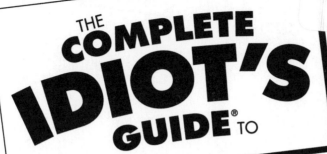

Glycemic Index Weight Loss

Second Edition

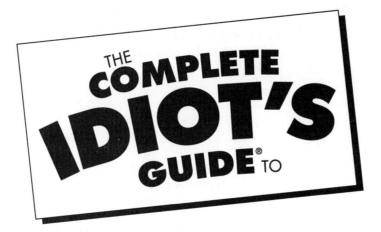

THE **COMPLETE IDIOT'S GUIDE®** TO

Glycemic Index Weight Loss

Second Edition

*by Lucy Beale and
Joan Clark-Warner, M.S., R.D., C.D.E.*

ALPHA

A member of Penguin Group (USA) Inc.

Lucy: To my husband, Patrick
Joan: To my husband, Douglas

ALPHA BOOKS

Published by the Penguin Group

Penguin Group (USA) Inc., 375 Hudson Street, New York, New York 10014, USA

Penguin Group (Canada), 90 Eglinton Avenue East, Suite 700, Toronto, Ontario M4P 2Y3, Canada (a division of Pearson Penguin Canada Inc.)

Penguin Books Ltd., 80 Strand, London WC2R 0RL, England

Penguin Ireland, 25 St. Stephen's Green, Dublin 2, Ireland (a division of Penguin Books Ltd.)

Penguin Group (Australia), 250 Camberwell Road, Camberwell, Victoria 3124, Australia (a division of Pearson Australia Group Pty. Ltd.)

Penguin Books India Pvt. Ltd., 11 Community Centre, Panchsheel Park, New Delhi—110 017, India

Penguin Group (NZ), 67 Apollo Drive, Rosedale, North Shore, Auckland 1311, New Zealand (a division of Pearson New Zealand Ltd.)

Penguin Books (South Africa) (Pty.) Ltd., 24 Sturdee Avenue, Rosebank, Johannesburg 2196, South Africa

Penguin Books Ltd., Registered Offices: 80 Strand, London WC2R 0RL, England

International Standard Book Number: 978-1-59257-855-9
Library of Congress Catalog Card Number: 2008933151

12 11 10   8 7 6 5 4 3 2 1

Interpretation of the printing code: The rightmost number of the first series of numbers is the year of the book's printing; the rightmost number of the second series of numbers is the number of the book's printing. For example, a printing code of 10-1 shows that the first printing occurred in 2010.

Printed in the United States of America

Note: This publication contains the opinions and ideas of its authors. It is intended to provide helpful and informative material on the subject matter covered. It is sold with the understanding that the authors and publisher are not engaged in rendering professional services in the book. If the reader requires personal assistance or advice, a competent professional should be consulted.

The authors and publisher specifically disclaim any responsibility for any liability, loss, or risk, personal or otherwise, which is incurred as a consequence, directly or indirectly, of the use and application of any of the contents of this book.

Most Alpha books are available at special quantity discounts for bulk purchases for sales promotions, premiums, fundraising, or educational use. Special books, or book excerpts, can also be created to fit specific needs.

For details, write: Special Markets, Alpha Books, 375 Hudson Street, New York, NY 10014.

Publisher: *Marie Butler-Knight*
Editorial Director: *Mike Sanders*
Senior Managing Editor: *Billy Fields*
Acquisitions Editor: *Michele Wells*
Development Editor: *Nancy D. Lewis*
Senior Production Editor: *Janette Lynn*

Copy Editor: *Michael Dietsch*
Cover Designer: *Rebecca Harmon*
Book Designer: *Trina Wurst*
Indexer: *Angie Bess*
Layout: *Ayanna Lacey*
Proofreader: *Laura Caddell*

Contents at a Glance

Contents

Appendixes

Introduction

Losing weight by eating based on the glycemic index is scientifically based and quite simple. We consider it almost a miracle. It's easy to use, socially below the radar, and eliminates many unpleasant dieting traditions, such as counting calories and restaurant ordering complications. Glycemic index eating is recommended by many health practitioners; you'll lose weight while improving your health. Dieting and deprivation will become phantoms of your past as you enjoy eating luscious, glycemic index–savvy meals that make your excess pounds melt away.

In this book, you learn the why and how of glycemic index weight loss—why it works and how to follow an eating plan that works for you. Our book discusses two approaches to eating based on the glycemic index that are doable and practical: the Keep It Simple Program, and the Comprehensive Program.

In this revised edition, we've added the Glycemic Index Food Source Guide and techniques for creating a flatter tummy among other tips. You'll learn how to manage the stress, insulin, and cortisol interactions associated with past high-glycemic eating and recover your nutritional balance with low-glycemic eating. You'll read about simple ways to turn exercise into your weight-loss friend for lifelong enjoyment.

If you've chosen this book because you want to reach your ideal size, you're ready to succeed. With the information in this book, you can synchronize the full force of your commitment, energy, and lifestyle with your weight-loss goals. The synergy that results is sure to make you a winner of the weight-loss challenge!

How This Book Is Organized

This book is divided into six parts:

Part 1, "All About the Glycemic Index," gives you a solid scientific and biological understanding of glycemic index weight loss. You learn how the glycemic index was first created when researchers realized that not all carbohydrates affect blood sugar and insulin levels in the same way. The glycemic index aids in weight loss, reducing insulin resistance, and boosting metabolism.

Part 2, "Designing Your Glycemic Index Weight-Loss Program," offers you a choice of two different programs, Keep It Simple and Comprehensive, for attaining your weight-loss goals. You'll learn how to eat based on the Glycemic Index Food Source Guide and how to set goals you can meet.

Part 3, "Nutritionally Balanced Eating," shows you the value of proteins, fats, and dairy for your glycemic index weight-loss program. Learn how to deal with sugars and junk foods, plus learn important information on which nutritional supplements can enhance your weight-loss program.

Part 4, "Eating for All Occasions," gives you valuable suggestions for eating based on the glycemic index at home, at parties, and even while traveling and vacationing. You learn how to shop for groceries and how to plan low-glycemic meals.

Part 5, "Insulin, Cortisol, and Weight Loss," offers new information on the biological interactions between insulin and the stress hormone, cortisol. By keeping your stress levels low, you can enhance your weight-loss progress. We show you how.

Part 6, "The Exercise Advantage," shows you how the three types of exercise—aerobic, strength training, and stretching—help you reduce insulin resistance and manage stress. Exercise does more than help your weight-loss efforts by burning through calories; it actually changes your biology.

Extras

We know you don't own a secret decoder ring to help you in the confusing world of glycemic index weight loss—and you shouldn't have to. This book has a few easy-to-recognize signposts that offer tips, tricks, and tidbits to help you along the way. Look for these elements in this book that will point you in the right direction:

Glyco Lingo
With these definitions you'll be in-the-know about the science, biology, and technicalities of glycemic index weight loss.

THIN-couragement
Use these helpful tips and hints as your personal coach for achieving your weight-loss goals.

Body of Knowledge
Gain the knowledge and dietary background about glycemic index eating you need so that you can better master your eating and your weight.

Wrong Weigh
Watch out! Avoid these glycemic index eating pitfalls so that you don't falter, but instead gain self-confidence and self-assurance with every bite.

Acknowledgments

Lucy and Joan give special thanks to their clients and friends, without whom they wouldn't have gleaned the special hands-on information and practical suggestions that are added into every page of this book.

Lucy Beale thanks her husband, Patrick, for his patience and support while she was occupied and preoccupied with writing. She also thanks her stepson, Stephen, for timely grammar and editing assistance. Lucy thanks her co-author, Joan, for her thoughtful, scientific expertise, as well as her insightful comments and suggestions.

Joan Clark-Warner thanks her husband, Douglas, for his patience and kindness; and her children, Jenny, Ryan, and Tricia, for their encouragement. Joan thanks the author, Lucy, for her expertise, enthusiasm, and creativity.

Lucy and Joan both thank Marilyn Allen of the Allen O'Shea Literary Agency and Michele Wells, acquisitions editor at Alpha Books, for guiding this book from inception through publication. Special thanks to Jennie Brand-Miller for permission to excerpt the glycemic index from her book, *What Makes My Blood Glucose Go Up ... And Down?* written with Kaye Foster-Powell and Rick Mendosa. And to Rick Mendosa for creating www.mendosa.com, which offers valuable and practical information on the glycemic index.

Special Thanks to the Technical Reviewer

The Complete Idiot's Guide to Glycemic Index Weight Loss, Second Edition, was reviewed by an expert who double-checked the accuracy of what you'll learn here, to help us ensure that this book gives you everything you need to know about losing weight using the glycemic index. Special thanks are extended to Lisa Vislocky.

Trademarks

All terms mentioned in this book that are known to be or are suspected of being trademarks or service marks have been appropriately capitalized. Alpha Books and Penguin Group (USA) Inc. cannot attest to the accuracy of this information. Use of a term in this book should not be regarded as affecting the validity of any trademark or service mark.

Part 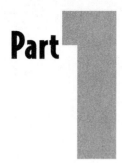 All About the Glycemic Index

Glycemic index weight loss isn't a "fad," and for good reason. It's a highly regarded and scientifically validated method for significant and successful weight loss. It's also a way to eat to improve your health and reduce the risk of chronic health conditions.

Glycemic index weight loss lowers insulin levels and insulin resistance, increases energy, and even lowers stress. As your body stops storing fat, you begin to burn fat for energy while you boost your metabolism. Thus you lose weight.

The glycemic index used hand-in-hand with the glycemic load will have you eating plenty of healthy, nutrient-dense carbohydrates—especially ones containing phytonutrients, antioxidants, vitamins, minerals, and dietary fiber.

The Glycemic Index: An Amazing Weight-Loss Tool

In This Chapter

- ◆ Appreciating how the glycemic index is different
- ◆ Managing blood sugar levels
- ◆ Learning about scientific research studies
- ◆ Accepting the glycemic index worldwide

If you've heard of the glycemic index, you may have already begun to use it as a guide for eating and for weight loss. Good for you. If you haven't heard about it, you're in for a treat—and not just the kind of treat you eat. Instead, it's the kind of treat that makes losing weight easy and knowing what to eat fail-proof.

The glycemic index is just plain brilliant because it's based on the science of how foods, specifically carbohydrates, work in your body. But the glycemic index isn't merely someone's good idea or an interesting intellectual theory. The glycemic index has been research-tested on real people, just like you, for over 20 years. These people have the same kinds of weight-loss and health issues as you. That's how we know it works.

Beyond Other Diets

Glycemic index weight loss goes beyond any diet program you've ever tried and does what all the other programs have tried to do. For starters, it explains why you've gained weight from both biological and behavioral points of view. It teaches you how to eat adequate amounts of delicious healthy food. It keeps your body from storing new fat by keeping your *blood sugar levels* and *insulin levels* within normal range. It even lets you eat treat foods from time to time without gaining weight.

Perhaps you've tried some of the diets listed below. Here's why they don't work long-term:

- **Strict low-carbohydrate diets.** They encourage you to eat large quantities of meats and fats, while limiting vegetables and fruits. Overeating all by itself encourages *insulin resistance*, which leads to weight gain.

- **Extreme low-fat diets.** Your body needs about 20 to 30 percent of your calories from fat intake per day to maintain good health and enjoy having healthy hair, skin, nails, muscles, and joints. This percentage range allows you to ingest adequate amounts of the essential fatty acids. Without adequate good fats, your body can't release stored fat. Plus, extremely low-fat diets encourage people to eat lots of low-fat, processed foods that are usually high in high-glycemic carbohydrates. Eating high-glycemic carbohydrates leads to insulin resistance and weight gain.

- **Extreme low-calorie diets.** Because they disregard the balance of the nutrients you need, they can be unhealthy. A dieter can stay within the limited calorie restrictions by eating too many high-glycemic foods, and the weight-loss results will be disappointing. It isn't healthy to eat less than 1,200 calories a day. This is the bare minimum amount of calories most people will need to obtain an adequate amount of nutrients to stay healthy and prevent *starvation metabolism*. Indirectly, a low-calorie diet can lead to insulin resistance and weight gain.

- **Fad diets.** Diets such as the cabbage-soup diet, the liquid diet, or food combining aren't based on scientific research and biological studies. As such, they don't offer safe and reliable long-term weight loss. Plus, they don't offer a reasonable approach to lifelong healthy eating, and they do not encourage a balanced diet supplying people with adequate vitamins and minerals.

Glyco Lingo _____

Blood sugar levels are considered healthy when the fasting level is between 70 and 120. Healthy **insulin levels** are between 4 and 27. To find your blood glucose or your insulin levels, check with your physician.

Insulin resistance occurs when there is a decrease in the ability of the body's cells to readily uptake glucose for energy. In other words, insulin can no longer effectively transport glucose into the cells. This condition can occur more readily when one is overweight and as one ages. In addition, some individuals could have more insulin resistance due to their genetic makeup.

Starvation metabolism occurs when a person doesn't eat enough calories on a day-to-day basis to sustain normal metabolic functioning. A person's body then conserves energy by slowing down most metabolic processes, which can include fat-burning—just what you don't want to happen.

♦ **Yo-yo dieting.** Losing weight, then regaining, and then losing the same pounds over and over again makes it increasingly difficult for a person to lose weight permanently. Basically, yo-yo dieting messes with your metabolism and keeps you overweight regardless of your best efforts. But don't despair—eating low glycemic over time can restore a burned-out metabolism.

Body of Knowledge _____

Is the glycemic index just another fad? The answer is a resounding No! It's a medically sound, scientifically tested explanation for how the body reacts to the foods we eat. The glycemic index has been used since the 1980s and today is used by nutritionists around the world to guide people—especially those with eating challenges, such as persons with diabetes and obesity.

While this is true, it is also a controversial topic because the GI of different foods can vary dramatically depending on preparation method and ripeness of a fruit or vegetable. So it is a guide for healthier eating, and a life saver for diabetics, but not always a promise of many other things for otherwise healthy people.

Weight loss by eating lower glycemic index carbohydrates keeps your insulin levels normal and reduces insulin resistance, allowing you to lose weight steadily and safely while eating plenty of food. You definitely won't go hungry while following a glycemic index weight-loss program. In all fairness, we should mention that you won't be eating stacks of donuts, muffins, or bagels any more. You can, however, eat them sometimes. Besides, you probably weren't eating them—except on the sly—on any other program either.

Glycemic Index for You

With this book in your hand, you have the power to lose weight safely and assuredly. Plus, the glycemic index can improve your overall health, maintain lean muscle mass, and balance your moods.

That's a big claim for anything, let alone something as fundamentally simple as the glycemic index. But you'll soon understand why it's true. The basic simplicity of it is one of its strengths.

Using the glycemic index picks up where other diet programs end. Strict low-carbohydrate diet programs tend to leave you hungry, cranky, and feeling deprived, which makes them hard to maintain in the long-term. Other programs that require restricting calories, drinking meal-replacement shakes, and eating prepackaged meals tend to leave you feeling that "eating's no fun anymore." That's not good and it creates a rebound effect.

Before we tell you exactly what using the glycemic index is all about, first let us tell you what it's not:

- ◆ **It's not a starvation program.** You'll be able to eat plenty of food throughout the day and not end up ravenous in the late afternoon. You'll eat a balanced diet of carbohydrates, fats, and proteins.

- ◆ **It doesn't include diet phases.** You won't need to endure a two-week induction phase or a special maintenance phase. The same program you start with is the one you will continue to use throughout your life.

- ◆ **It doesn't include special diet foods.** You won't need to purchase contrived specialty diet foods. Instead, you'll eat wholesome, commonly available foods. You could end up making a couple trips to the health-food store for some whole grains or sweeteners, but most of your food supply can come from your neighborhood grocery store.

- ◆ **It doesn't contain artificial foods.** You won't need to use any controversial foods, such as aspartame, sucralose, *trans-fats* or other highly processed packaged foods.

As you can tell, using the glycemic index is unlike any diet program you've ever tried. You won't find gimmicks. Instead you'll eat the types of food that let you lose weight and keep it off.

Here's what using the glycemic index for weight loss offers you:

- **Wholesome and delicious foods that are readily available and highly satisfying.** You can be a gourmet cook or a person who prefers to eat prepared foods or one who dines out frequently, and you'll still be able to use the glycemic index.

- **Reduced food cravings.** Of course, you may still want that special piece of chocolate or slice of bread, and you can eat it occasionally without guilt.

- **Energy maintenance.** Helps maintaining balanced energy levels throughout the day so you avoid late-afternoon energy slumps.

- **Helps reducing stress by lowering *cortisol levels*.** The kinds of food you eat actually help reduce stress. High cortisol levels lead to weight gain, so keeping your stress levels low is a big benefit.

> **Glyco Lingo** _____
>
> **Trans-fatty acids** come from liquid fats that have been changed by food processors by adding hydrogen molecules. Trans-fatty acids are also known as hydrogenated and partially hydrogenated oils. They don't occur in natural foods except in very small amounts.
>
> **Cortisol levels** are high when a person's short- or long-term stress is high. Recent studies suggest a positive association between elevated cortisol levels and the risk of such chronic conditions as weight gain, diabetes, heart disease, cancer, and high blood pressure.

- **Some treat foods.** You can factor in your favorite treats to your daily food intake and enjoy eating them while still losing weight.

- **The kinds of food you eat when you lose weight are the same foods you'll eat after you've attained your ideal size.** You can stick with low- and moderate-glycemic eating for life.

- **Improved health.** Low-glycemic eating improves overall health and reduces the risk or the reality of chronic disease conditions.

- **Lifestyle friendly.** No diet should force you to live your life constantly worrying about finding and eating "special foods." That's not our definition of *special*. Unlike many diets, using the glycemic index is lifestyle-friendly. It influences the foods you eat, but it never makes eating seem unpleasant or depressing.

Information about eating based on the glycemic index is now widely available. You'll find information on the Internet and in some popular diet books. We predict that the popularity of the glycemic index is only beginning and will last for a very long time. Your choice of using the glycemic index as a basis for eating and weight loss is a wise and sound decision.

Glycemic Index Basics

Before you can delve into the exquisite and elegant weight-loss resources of the glycemic index, you need to know the basics of what it is and what it means.

Here's a simple definition: the *glycemic index* is a scientific measurement of how a person's blood sugar levels change after eating different types of carbohydrate foods. The glycemic index's ranking system is only for carbohydrates and not for proteins or fats.

By itself, the glycemic index isn't an eating program; it's just a way of understanding the impact of carbohydrates on the body. But it is critical for following a healthy eating program. Initially the index was used as a guide for persons with diabetes to help keep their blood sugar levels in the healthy range. Since then, it's been used for weight loss and weight management.

Body of Knowledge

Although the glycemic index is used to measure how carbohydrates affect blood sugar levels, the amount of proteins and fats you eat with carbohydrates can affect blood sugar levels in the body. They're intertwined. High blood sugar levels can ultimately cause weight gain. You'll learn more later in this chapter.

A Brief History

During the 1980s the very low-fat diet craze took hold, and people were encouraged by health and nutrition experts to eat lots of grains, pastas, and breads—high-glycemic carbohydrates—whether processed or not, while keeping their fat intake very low. For many individuals the approach backfired. High-carb, especially if it is of the high-glycemic variety, proved to be especially detrimental to persons with diabetes. While eating low fat, they weren't able to maintain stable blood sugar levels because they were eating too many high-glycemic foods; and to make matters worse, they gained weight. Persons with diabetes weren't alone. The high-carb, very low-fat approach to eating added many extra inches to the waists of countless individuals. Eating about

20 to 30 percent of your diet as fat is now considered eating low fat in a healthy way and is recommended in this book.

Body of Knowledge

Type 2 diabetes is a serious problem in the United States and worldwide. Today, many children and young adults have type 2 diabetes due to poor diet and lack of exercise. To stay healthy, persons with diabetes need to keep their blood sugar levels stable and within the normal range of about 70 to 120. Most of the time they can do this through diet, exercise, or oral medications. However, if their pancreatic cells have "worn out" due to years of overstimulation of the pancreas, they may need insulin-based injections. In most cases, type 2 diabetics still can produce insulin, but their body cells can't use it adequately. Their cells have become "insulin resistant." Insulin resistance becomes worse as a person gets older and also becomes worse if the person is over-weight. This is true of persons with type 2 diabetes, and for everyone.

In type 1 diabetes, the pancreatic cells are damaged and consequently produce inadequate amounts or no insulin.

During the low-fat/high-carb phase, Thomas M. S. Wolever, M.D., Ph.D., a professor in the Department of Nutritional Sciences at the University of Toronto in Canada, began conducting research on the effect of carbohydrates on a person's blood sugar levels. His studies were focused on people with type 2 diabetes, which is often known as adult-onset diabetes.

In his research, Dr. Wolever found that some carbohydrates increased blood sugar levels to a greater degree than other carbohydrates. He wanted to discover which foods helped keep blood sugar levels more stable. His explorations led him to design a method for measuring the blood sugar–raising effect of different carbohydrates. The glycemic index was born.

Soon Jennie Brand-Miller, Ph.D., a professor at the University of Sydney in Australia, joined in the research. She has written a whole series of books in the Glucose Revolution series.

Their research and publications have helped thousands and thousands of people control their diabetes through diet. But the value of their research has extended far beyond that to people who want to lose weight and others who want increased good health.

In the past decade, eating mostly low glycemic has been shown to benefit persons with autoimmune disorders, heart disease, high cholesterol, high blood pressure, obesity, allergies, anxiety, depression, mood disorders, and high stress.

The glycemic index as a basis of dietary and nutritional requirements is widely accepted among health professionals and dietitians in Canada and Australia. Although the United States medical community has been slow to formally recognize the glycemic index, many health-care practitioners now recommend it to their patients. It's also mentioned and recommended in many of the most popular diet books, including *Sugar Busters!*, *The Zone*, *The South Beach Diet*, and *The New Atkins Diet Revolution*.

Experimental Findings

The glycemic index has excellent credibility and scientific validity because it's been experimentally tested on people—lots of people. Here's a brief overview of how the testing was done and how the glycemic index scale was set up.

Researchers used pure glucose as a baseline standard for the effect that carbohydrates have on blood sugar. First, the blood sugar levels of the research volunteers were tested. Then the volunteers were given glucose to drink. Yes, pure glucose. Although not something found in the average kitchen pantry, glucose is a thick and sweet, though palatable, liquid. About a half-hour later, blood sugar levels were retested. The difference in blood sugar levels told the researchers the amount of glucose needed to cause a rise in blood sugar.

The researchers then arbitrarily set the glycemic index of glucose to 100. This established a reference with which to analyze other foods. The researchers started testing other carbohydrates on their volunteers. They discovered wildly different effects based on the food. The glycemic index of carbohydrates tested ranged widely, from almost 0 to 115.

Body of Knowledge

Carbs of all sorts have been given "scores" on the glycemic index. Some lettuces are very low on the glycemic index and are given a glycemic index rank of 0. The highest-ranking carb is a tofu frozen dessert at 115.

By using the glycemic index as a reference when you eat, you actually know how a food will affect your weight and health. With many food theories, such as food combining or vegetarian eating, personal testimonials are often the only evidence. And these are often based on a person's internal belief systems, motivation, and perhaps a desire to prove a point (or not). With actual testing, well, let's put it this way—it would have been difficult and most likely impossible for a volunteer to fool the blood sugar/glucose test.

Research Methods

Early testing of the glycemic effect was a bit inconsistent, but methods for determining the glycemic index of a food have become standardized. Consequently, some early glycemic index lists are now out-of-date and have been revised.

An early test indicated that carrots were high glycemic. When you think about this, it doesn't make sense. All vegetables are low glycemic, so why would carrots be high? Recent standardized testing puts cooked carrots at 47 and raw carrot juice at 43. Both are low glycemic, and this makes more sense.

Here's how the testing is now done. Foods are tested on groups of eight to ten people. They consume a standard serving of a carbohydrate in 10 to 15 minutes. A blood sample is taken before the meal and every 15 minutes after for one hour. Then one is taken every 30 minutes for the next hour. Results are entered into a computer for analysis.

At another time, the volunteers do the same test, but this time with pure glucose, because pure glucose provides the baseline for the glycemic index. Pure glucose is 100. The computer analyzes the results, giving a value for the food tested based on the value compared to 100.

The glycemic index of any carbohydrate is an average of the effect on the individuals tested. The real change in blood sugar levels of a specific carbohydrate varies by person, but the variations follow the pattern established by the index. In other words, it's reliable.

The glycemic index value of a specific food can vary due to food preparation methods and the ripeness of fruits and vegetables. Glycemic index charts account for this variation by averaging results for each food. The range of variations is usually small and not significant for weight loss.

Classifications of Carbohydrates

As you know from previous dieting experiences, carbohydrates are present in a wide variety of foods. The glycemic index has been used to develop a very comprehensive list that ranks virtually all the available edible carbohydrates. The sources of carbohydrates are the following:

- ◆ **Starches.** This group includes all foods made from starches, such as bread, flour, oatmeal, breakfast cereals, tortillas, cookies, pasta, pizza, donuts, and muffins.

Starches can be refined or unrefined. In addition to processed, manmade starchy foods, white and sweet potatoes, yams, corn, rice, and winter squash are starchy.

◆ **Sugars.** Including naturally occurring honey and molasses, plus table sugar, fruit sugar (called fructose), and milk sugars (called lactose and galactose). Natural sweeteners include sugar alcohols, such as xylitol and mannitol. High-fructose corn syrup (HFCS) is a sweetener commonly used in packaged foods, sodas, juice beverages, and electrolyte-replenishment drinks. Also included in the sugar category are shakes, lattes, cappuccinos, and other beverages that contain one of these types of sweetener. Candy and candy bars are in the sugar category.

◆ **Fruits.** This category includes all fruit, from apples and pears to pineapple, watermelon, and pomegranate, and fruit juices.

◆ **Vegetables.** This category contains all vegetables, from lettuces and radishes to summer squash and carrots.

◆ **Nuts and seeds.** These are combination foods. They contain mostly fat, but also some carbohydrates and protein. Nuts and seeds that don't contain any net carbohydrates, such as pecans and macadamia nuts, aren't tested, because their GI is zero. Two exceptions are cashews and peanuts (actually a legume), as they do contain enough carbohydrates to be tested. Both are low glycemic.

THIN-couragement

Even though watermelon is high glycemic, it consists of more water and air than carbs so its glycemic load isn't high. It's a healthy food and contains vitamins, minerals, and antioxidants, so go ahead and enjoy eating watermelon, but eat in moderation, meaning no more than one cup per day.

◆ **Dairy products.** This category includes milk, yogurt, and ice milk. Usually dairy products contain fat and animal protein. Cheese isn't included here as a dairy product because it contains no carbohydrates or very few. Cheese is considered a protein.

◆ **Legumes.** Lentils, soy, peanuts, and pinto beans are carbohydrates. Peanuts are considered to be a fat, but they also contain some carbohydrate, and their glycemic index is low at 14.

Many foods contain combinations of the previous categories, and the glycemic index of many processed foods and combination foods are available. See Appendix B for information on where to find glycemic index values for most foods.

High, Medium, and Low

After researchers created a baseline by assigning glucose a value of 100, they assigned a score to all the other carbohydrates, either higher or lower than 100. Carbohydrates with a glycemic index of 55 or lower are considered low glycemic; those from 56 to 69 are medium glycemic; those 70 or higher are high glycemic. You'll find a comprehensive listing of the glycemic index of foods in Appendix B, but here are some general guidelines:

♦ Some cookies have high-glycemic values, and some have mid-level values. Ice cream can be middle or low, depending on the ingredients used. The glycemic index values for these kinds of products vary. They vary based on methods of cooking, and the amounts of flour, sugar, butter, and other ingredients used. That's why it's best to check with a glycemic index list before you eat.

♦ High-glycemic foods include breads, rice crackers, some cookies and cakes, most muffins, and most foods made with enriched white or wheat flour. The more easily digestible the starches and sugars in a food, the higher it is on the glycemic index. Refined grain products are usually high as well as most breakfast cereals, white potatoes, and modified food starch. The only fruit that's high glycemic is watermelon and its value is 72.

♦ Medium-glycemic foods include stone-ground breads that don't contain white flour, whole-grain cereals, some cakes and cookies, corn taco shells, table sugar, and energy bars. Some tropical fruits, such as papaya and pineapple, are medium glycemic.

♦ Low-glycemic foods include all vegetables, most fruits, some whole-grain products such as steel-cut oats and whole barley, and *al dente* pasta. Legumes, such as lentils and pinto beans, are low glycemic. Dark chocolate is, too, with a glycemic index of 48. Nuts and seeds are low or 0, and most dairy products, provided they don't have added sugar, are also low.

Wrong Weigh _____

Some foods, such as honey and rice, vary in their glycemic index value. Some varieties of rice are high, some are low, and some are medium. The same is true for honey. The tested values differ based on where the foods were produced, what varieties were tested, and other factors we don't yet fully understand.

In your weight-loss program based on the glycemic index, you'll eat carbohydrates that are high, medium, and low glycemic, but you'll mostly eat the ones that are low.

The Least You Need to Know

- ◆ The glycemic index was developed in the 1980s as a way to quantify how carbohydrates affect blood-sugar levels.

- ◆ Eating in alignment with the glycemic index promotes improved health, lower blood sugar levels, and weight loss.

- ◆ The glycemic index is receiving recognition worldwide, but has been slower to catch on in the United States with nutritionists, dietitians, and medical practitioners.

- ◆ Carbohydrates are broadly categorized by the glycemic index as high, medium, or low glycemic.

2

The Glycemic Index and Insulin Levels

In This Chapter

◆ Benefiting from carbohydrates

◆ Learning the dynamics of carbohydrates and insulin

◆ Pairing stress with insulin

◆ Having high insulin levels can cause health conditions

Carbohydrates are a fascinating category of food. You've been told for years to eat your vegetables, which are low-glycemic carbohydrates and superbly good for you. Most high-glycemic foods are the comfort and treat foods that lead to cravings, overeating, and weight gain. Don't give them up—that's too hard. Instead eat them sparingly and budget them into your meal plans. That way, you can still eat some birthday or wedding cake, some ballpark snacks, and such foods as pretzels or chips from time to time.

In this chapter, you learn more about how your carbohydrate consumption relates directly to your weight and your health. By understanding the health risks associated with eating high-glycemic foods, you will strengthen your resolve to attain your ideal size and maintain it.

Health-Giving Carbohydrates

Every day, newspapers, the Internet, and television applaud the health benefits of fruits and vegetables. You're advised to eat 5 to 10 servings a day. That seems like a lot but actually is less than you might think. A serving for nonstarchy vegetables, such as broccoli, is one cup uncooked or ½ cup cooked. A serving for fruit is generally ½ cup or four ounces.

When eating your daily 5 to 10 servings of vegetables and fruits—think 2 to 3 per meal—be sure to keep from overloading on carbohydrates, that is, from having too high a *glycemic load*. You'll learn more about the glycemic load in Chapter 5. But for now, know that eating five servings of fruit at one sitting is too high a glycemic load. So is eating five servings of starchy vegetables, such as legumes, winter squash, sweet potatoes, corn, and lima beans, all at one sitting.

There are good reasons nutritionists and dietitians recommend you eat low-glycemic carbohydrates. Vegetables and fruits are the basis of a healthy diet. In addition to dietary fiber, plant foods, including nuts and seeds, provide important *phytonutrients*.

Glyco Lingo

Glycemic load is a calculation of the amount of a carbohydrate food factored by the glycemic index of the food. This number gives you a good sense of how what you eat will affect your blood sugar levels and insulin levels. It lets you predict what effect a serving of a carbohydrate food will have on your blood sugar levels.

Phytonutrients are plant-derived essential nutrients scientifically confirmed as important to human health. They are found in plants and plant products, such as vegetables, fruits, nuts, and seeds.

Most vegetables are low glycemic. Most fruits are low glycemic, some are medium glycemic, and only a few like watermelon are high glycemic.

In the information that follows, you'll learn about the nutritional goodness found in vegetables and fruits.

Fiber

You need to consume between 25 to 45 grams of dietary fiber every day. Fiber increases the transit time of food in the digestive system, keeps your bowel movements regular, keeps your LDL cholesterol low, and helps remove toxins from your body quickly.

A fast transit time of food reduces the risk of colon cancer. Fiber also gives you a sense of satiation when you eat that helps prevent overeating. But wait, there's even more good news about fiber! Eating foods high in fiber can reduce the effective glycemic index of your meal. And the more fiber in the food, the lower the glycemic index. That's one of the reasons that true stone-ground breads are generally lower than white bread in the glycemic index.

Whole-wheat breads and some stone-ground breads can be high glycemic because in addition to the coarsely milled flour, they contain finely milled flour or added sugars. The more finely milled the flour, the faster your stomach digests it, causing a faster rise in blood sugar levels. Purchase breads that are heavy in weight rather than fluffy and that have rough-ground grains. Make sure the label contains just a few ingredients—stone-ground flour, yeast, water, salt, and not much more.

> **Wrong Weigh** _____
>
> Although some people may try to receive the full nutritional value of vegetables and fruits by taking dietary supplements, research indicates that it's best to actually consume these gifts from the garden rather than bypass their innate goodness by simply swallowing pills. Think of vitamin, mineral, and antioxidant supplements as nutritional insurance. You can certainly take them but, as your mom always said, "Eat your vegetables!"

Try this little imaginary experiment. Picture yourself hungry and gobbling down a half dozen glazed donuts in just a couple of minutes, but then not feeling "satisfied" 20 minutes later. Plausible, right? Now imagine trying to eat an amount of high-fiber celery that contains a comparable total carbohydrate count. Guess how much that would be? You would need to eat more than 90 cups of diced celery to equal the total carb count of 6 donuts! You would feel full after about 20 minutes of eating celery and still have about three days' worth of chewing to go! The lesson: high-fiber carbs with low-carb counts fit into a healthy diet.

So eat foods high in fiber. And only carbohydrates contain fiber. Neither fats nor animal proteins, such as meat, seafood, dairy, eggs, and cheese, contain fiber. You can take a fiber supplement, such as psyllium, to increase your fiber intake. But don't skimp on foods that contain naturally occurring fiber such as fruits and vegetables. They add a variety of different types of fiber and increase stomach satisfaction with meals. You also get the extra benefit of the nutrients consumed. Take a fiber supplement one half hour away from meals, medications, or supplements, because the additional fiber can block absorption of some nutrients and medications.

Vitamins and Minerals

Consider vegetables and fruits to be your vitamin and mineral warehouse. The water-soluble vitamins, such as vitamin C and the B vitamins, need to be replenished daily because they are either used or flushed from the body continuously. Your body doesn't store these vitamins. This is why you need to eat a variety of vegetables and fruits daily. B vitamins are also present in meat, eggs, and other animal protein, so you obtain them when you eat your moderate serving of animal proteins.

Not all vitamins are water soluble. Vitamins A, D, E, and K are not. They're stored in fat in the body. One or more fat-soluble vitamins are found in nuts, seeds, fish, meats, poultry, eggs, some vegetables, grains, and oils. Vitamin D is present in cod-liver oil and is manufactured on your skin when exposed to sunshine.

> **Glyco Lingo**
>
> Major minerals are those that our bodies need daily in at least an amount of 100 mg (1/50 of a teaspoon). All other minerals are considered to be **trace minerals** because the body only needs very small amounts of them.

Your body needs a plethora of minerals. The primary ones are calcium, potassium, and magnesium. Your body also needs *trace minerals* such as zinc, iron, chromium, copper, vanadium, manganese, phosphorous, molybdenum, lithium, cadmium, and boron. (Added all together, it sounds like just about every element from the periodic chart in high school chemistry!) You can find them in the vegetables you eat, as well as from animal protein. You may not need more than tiny amounts of some of the trace elements, but without them, your body's metabolic processes won't work as well.

Antioxidants

Discoveries of new antioxidants occur almost weekly. Once virtually unknown, antioxidants are now front-page news. They protect our bodies from the ravages of free radicals. These free radicals can wreak havoc on bodily functions and our immune systems. Damage from free radicals has been implicated in cancer, mood disorders, degenerative diseases, and even wrinkled skin.

Vegetables and fruits are filled with healthful antioxidants, such as carotenoids, flavonoids, coumarins, phenolic acids, bioflavonoids, lycopene, and many more. You will also find antioxidants in many popular spices, coffee, tea, and herbs, which are also carbohydrates. Several nutritional supplements contain antioxidants, but you need to use them cautiously and not use the supplement to replace eating two to three servings of vegetables or fruit per meal.

Wrong Weigh

Antioxidant supplements sometimes work, but occasionally they actually create more free-radical damage. If you choose to take antioxidant supplements, first research the pros and cons of taking each antioxidant as a supplement. Be careful not to take more than the maximum amount recommended; too high an amount can be harmful.

A Gourmet Palate

Another very important advantage of eating your vegetables and fruits is that they make eating more interesting. A daily diet of only animal protein and fat would become boring in less than a day. But with vegetables, fruits, spices, and herbs, food becomes palatable, colorful, and tasty.

Just imagine food without sauces, without salsa, without condiments, without pesto. Such a dull life. Imagine no recipes, no garnishes, no pickles, and no ethnic cuisine. No one would even want to eat.

Carbohydrates save us from palate boredom. The varied fragrances whet our appetites and make mealtimes much more pleasurable. Hurrah for this aspect of carbs!

The Regulatory Hormone, Insulin

Insulin is a highly beneficial hormone. It literally keeps you alive. But again, too much of a good thing—in this case, insulin—is damaging. You want to have enough insulin circulating in your body to assist delivering glucose into body cells, but not so much that you unknowingly damage your body.

Insulin is the hormone that regulates blood sugar levels. It delivers energy in the form of glucose (sugar) to your body's cells. The beta cells of the pancreas gland secrete insulin in response to carbohydrate consumption. The higher the glycemic index of the carbohydrate, and the more you eat of it, the more insulin the pancreas pumps out. When you eat low-glycemic carbohydrates, the carbohydrates are digested more slowly and sugar enters the blood at a slower pace, and the pancreas secretes less insulin. Too much insulin in your bloodstream becomes a health problem and causes weight gain. Insulin is the body's fat-storing hormone, so you want to have enough, but not too much.

When your body has too much of this fat-storing hormone, it becomes inefficient at getting the cells to uptake glucose. This is the condition called insulin resistance.

♦ You eat too many high-glycemic carbohydrates. Insulin levels surge beyond what is needed by the body to adequately clear excess sugar from the blood. In the case of high-glycemic carbs, it doesn't take much to trigger too much insulin production. On the other hand, if you eat too many low-glycemic carbs—too high a glycemic load—you can also trigger too much insulin secretion. You'll learn how to balance your carb intake with the glycemic index of food in Chapter 5.

♦ You eat too high a *glycemic load* for a long period of time, as in months and years. Your body's cells become inefficient at responding to insulin, or insulin resistant, thus requiring the pancreas to produce more and more insulin to deliver sugar and fat to your cells for energy. You'll have excess insulin in your body that causes fat storage and weight gain.

♦ Your long-term stress levels are high. The stress hormone cortisol causes a corresponding increase in insulin.

♦ You are a person with type 2 diabetes or with impaired glucose tolerance, also known as borderline diabetes. Your body may no longer be able to efficiently uptake blood sugar into the cells. The body usually produces enough insulin, but your body cannot use the insulin well. Consequently, your blood sugar levels stay too high.

♦ You eat too much food. Continually overeating increases your insulin levels regardless of which food you're overeating. You can overproduce insulin by over-eating protein, fat, or carbohydrates.

♦ Fasting, not eating, or skipping meals can cause insulin resistance.

When you have too much insulin in your body, the excess insulin gives you low blood sugar and increases your stress level. This makes you lightheaded, jittery, and anxious while causing fatigue and sugar cravings.

Weight Gain

Insulin is the hormone that signals the body to store fat. When blood sugar levels surge, insulin signals for cell transporters to escort glucose into the cell. There, inside the cell, excess glucose is converted to triglycerides. Some of these triglycerides are moved into storage in your fat cells. And of course, you gain weight. Unfortunately, stored fat tends to stick around for a while.

By keeping your insulin levels balanced and avoiding insulin resistance, your body stops storing excess energy as fat. Instead your body uses your stored fat as fuel, and you lose weight. This occurs most efficiently on a low–glycemic index weight-loss program. Even after you lose weight and reach your ideal size, you need to avoid overstimulation of insulin production. Your maintenance phase requires that you focus on keeping your insulin levels balanced to avoid regaining weight.

Metabolic Syndrome

Metabolic syndrome is a condition that's considered a precursor to type 2 diabetes. It is also called Syndrome X. Read over the symptoms that follow. If you have these, chances are good that you have insulin resistance.

◆ Waist circumference over 40 inches in men and over 35 inches in women.

◆ High triglycerides of 150 milligrams per deciliter (mg/dL) or above.

◆ Low HDL cholesterol of 40 mg/dL or lower in men and 50 mg/dL or lower in women.

◆ Elevated blood pressure of 130/85 or more.

◆ High fasting blood glucose of 100 mg/dL or above.

If you know you have metabolic syndrome, you have a wonderful opportunity to halt its progression and to reduce its effects. Eat based on the glycemic index and exercise regularly and you'll enjoy lifetime benefits.

Type 2 Diabetes

Many people with type 2 diabetes also have elevated levels of insulin. Unfortunately, their insulin resistance prevents their bodies from efficiently delivering energy-giving sugars and fats to their cells. Their blood sugar levels can remain elevated. This leads to damaged blood vessels, which may cause eye disease, heart disease, early dementia, nerve damage to the limbs and internal organs, and kidney disease. In addition, persons with diabetes often continue to gain weight, leading to obesity, which brings its own set of health risks.

It's easy to see why a glycemic index weight-loss program is valuable and is recommended for individuals with type 2 diabetes and metabolic syndrome. It helps lower and stabilize blood sugar and insulin levels.

At your annual physical examination, ask your doctor to test for elevated blood sugar levels and elevated insulin levels. The sooner a person discovers he or she is at risk for type 2 diabetes, the easier it is to control the condition and avoid its debilitating consequences.

High LDL Cholesterol

In addition to increasing blood sugar, excess levels of insulin increase triglycerides. As a person gains weight, there's normally an increase in the *LDL* count. LDL is the so-called bad cholesterol. A high LDL count indicates a higher risk of heart attacks than a low LDL.

For many years health professionals believed that a diet high in *saturated fats* caused high cholesterol and heart disease. Now we know that the cause and effect is more complex. Eating lots of high-glycemic carbohydrates can cause elevated lipid levels and heart disease. Eating smaller amounts of high-glycemic carbohydrates and eating more low-glycemic carbohydrates boosts the good cholesterol (*HDL*).

> **Glyco Lingo**
>
> **LDL** is low-density lipoprotein and is called "bad" cholesterol. Keep your LDL levels below 100 mg/dL. **HDL** is high-density lipoprotein and is called "good" cholesterol. It's best if your levels of HDL are about 70 to 80 mg/dL and no lower than 35.
>
> **Saturated fats** have a molecular structure that is saturated with hydrogen atoms. Saturated fats are solid at room temperature. Butter and lard are saturated fats.

For the best results, limit the saturated fat in your diet, avoid all partially hydrogenated vegetable oils and trans-fats, eat meals that contain low-glycemic carbohydrates, keep your glycemic load within your goals, and drink alcoholic beverages sparingly if at all.

Thick Artery Walls

Elevated insulin levels cause the artery walls to grow thicker, which in effect narrows the diameter of the passageway. This makes it more likely that cholesterol will adhere inside the walls and lead to blocked arteries and heart disease.

As the passageways of the arteries get narrower, blood pressure increases, too.

Inflammation

Inflammation is another health-related consequence of elevated insulin levels. Many medical experts believe inflammation is a major cause of chronic disease. These diseases include cancer, Alzheimer's, acne, skin rashes, and autoimmune diseases such as allergies, asthma, fibromyalgia, multiple sclerosis, and arthritis. Even aging is thought to be a function of inflammation. (If this proves true, eating based on the glycemic index can become a veritable Fountain of Youth!)

)⅋ⅉ|ℕ -couragement

On a glycemic-savvy weight-loss program, you could lose several pounds of water weight in the first couple of weeks. This is good because it can help lower high blood pressure. Don't be concerned; you'll also be losing fat, and your fat loss will continue as your water weight stabilizes.

Research indicates that lowering insulin levels can help prevent inflammation and the resultant disease conditions. The best way to do that is to eat based on the glycemic index.

Magnesium Deficiency

Magnesium is a necessary mineral used by the body for more than 300 biochemical bodily functions. Some very important ones include relaxing the muscles, including the muscles of the arteries, improving insulin sensitivity, helping control blood pressure, and helping support the immune system.

It also eases muscle cramps. When insulin levels are elevated, the body stores less magnesium. This happens because insulin insensitivity affects the transport of magnesium as well as glucose into the cells. The more insulin resistance, the less magnesium gets through to the cells. Less magnesium in the body means that the blood vessels are more likely to be constricted, which leads to high blood pressure, and, further, it decreases the body's ability to regulate insulin.

It's a vicious cycle. When your body lacks adequate amounts of magnesium, you have less energy, which can lead to overeating and even binge eating. Eating foods that are low glycemic will enhance your intake of magnesium, because it enhances your insulin sensitivity. Whole, unprocessed grains and low-glycemic farm-sourced carbohydrates are high in many nutrients, including magnesium.

Polycystic Ovary Syndrome

When a woman's ovaries are exposed to too much insulin, polycystic ovary syndrome (PCOS) can occur. This leads to the ovaries producing too much of the hormones testosterone and androsterone. In the United States, 1 in 10 obese women have PCOS. It leads to hair loss, acne, and infertility and puts women at high risk for heart disease and type 2 diabetes.

The bottom line is that keeping your insulin levels in a normal range not only helps you lose weight and enjoy living at your ideal size, it definitely helps you stay healthy.

Skin Health

Having lots of wrinkles, sagging or puffy facial skin, and dark circles under the eyes hardly qualifies as a significant health problem, but perhaps as a significant self-esteem and social concern.

Research by dermatologists shows that people who eat low glycemic have better skin, fewer wrinkles, less puffiness, and lighter eye circles. Several factors play a role:

- Low-glycemic eating reduces overall inflammation.
- The high nutrient content of low-glycemic foods.
- Low-glycemic vegetables and fruit help protect your skin against sun damage.

To further increase your skin health, take essential fatty acids through diet or supplementation, avoid unprotected sun exposure, and don't smoke. Your skin will be positively radiant and glowing.

Stress and Insulin Levels

Adrenaline and cortisol are the "stress hormones." Your body produces these hormones to support your actions and thoughts when it feels under siege or threatened. This is good. But high levels of ongoing stress keep cortisol active in your body. And guess what? Too much cortisol for too long makes you gain weight. Insulin and cortisol are, in effect, team players. They need each other. When insulin levels are elevated, so are the levels of adrenaline and cortisol. The reverse is also true. When your stress levels are high, your insulin levels are elevated. When your insulin levels are balanced, your stress levels become balanced.

What this means is that you want to keep your stress levels low most of the time. Elevated stress levels contribute to health concerns:

◆ Cortisol overload causes weight gain in your midsection—the area around your waist and tummy.

◆ Cortisol overload breaks down muscle, causing your basal metabolic rate to slow down.

◆ Because cortisol overload reduces the number of muscle cells, a person has fewer cells to uptake blood sugar, so more sugar gets stored as fat, increasing body fat levels.

◆ Cortisol uses up brain chemicals, also known as neurotransmitters. When the brain neurotransmitter serotonin is depleted, a person can have difficulty sleeping and can feel depressed and anxious. These feelings in turn can lead to activities that further increase stress, such as smoking, drinking too much caffeine or alcoholic beverages, and eating high-glycemic comfort foods.

High stress always makes weight loss more difficult. If your stress levels are high, you may not be able to lose weight as quickly as you want, even on a glycemic-savvy weight-loss program. When you reduce your stress, you'll lose more quickly. In Chapter 23, you learn how to reduce stress and relax more so that you can keep your insulin levels low.

The Least You Need to Know

◆ Carbohydrates benefit your health by providing fiber, vitamins, minerals, and antioxidants.

◆ Elevated insulin levels cause weight gain and promote chronic health conditions and diseases.

◆ Carbohydrates provide appealing taste and color to meals and can delight the palate.

◆ A weight-loss program that is based on low-glycemic eating helps you lose weight and keep your insulin levels in a healthy range.

◆ High insulin levels from eating high-glycemic carbs increase the stress hormone cortisol, which can also lead to weight gain.

Glycemic Index Weight-Loss Benefits

In This Chapter

- ◆ Experiencing higher energy levels
- ◆ Reducing food cravings
- ◆ Managing your moods
- ◆ Having extra feel-good body perks
- ◆ Eating comfortably with others

Just the mention of the word *dieting* can bring back dreadful memories of past experiences and failures. If you dieted by reducing your caloric intake, you might have felt like you were starving. You probably tried valiantly to wrestle with and overcome your incredibly intense food cravings. You might also remember feeling bloated and constipated.

Stepping on scales occasionally gave you joyful highs but it more likely provoked self-doubt, lowered your self-esteem, and increased your anxiety. You, and others you loved, endured your dramatic and uncontrollable mood swings as your blood sugar levels plummeted midmorning and late afternoon. Of course, you were delighted when your clothes became looser and you could fit into a smaller pair of jeans—at least, temporarily—but you may have noticed that your appearance took on an unhealthy pallor.

The good news is that those dieting days are in your past. The "good old days" of deprivation dieting, when experts thought depriving yourself of food was the only way to lose weight, are over. With a glycemic index weight-loss program, you won't feel as if you're starving or suffering emotionally. In fact, you can lose weight while realizing terrific lifestyle and health benefits. In this chapter, you'll learn all about them.

Personal Gains

Glycemic index weight loss is exciting because it helps you feel good. Doesn't that just seem right? When you're doing good things for your body, such as losing weight, shouldn't you feel good throughout the entire process? Absolutely. Ideally, you should feel at least as good, if not better, than you feel when you aren't on a weight-loss program at all. That's what glycemic index weight loss has to offer!

With glycemic index weight loss, you can experience personal gains in day-to-day energy levels and drop pounds at the same time. You'll not only see the difference in how your clothes fit, you'll also notice a positive difference in the appearance of your skin, hair, and nails. You'll even find that your moods are brighter and more stable. And as an added bonus, your stress levels are likely to be reduced.

How is all this possible? Glycemic-savvy eating actually changes the way your body works.

Energy Levels

You want to have energy to burn, and you can. Your body already has abundant energy stored as fat. Glycemic index weight loss lets you access that stored fat and burn it for fuel. On many other kinds of diets, your body used both muscle and fat for energy. When you limit high-glycemic carbohydrate intake, however, your body uses up stored fat with less muscle loss.

All your excess weight is, in essence, stored energy, and with a glycemic index eating plan, you finally get to live off of your excess stored body fat and deplete it down to a healthy amount. You can't just stop eating and live entirely on stored fat. If you try this, you'll go into starvation metabolism and your body will conserve fat and store extra. But by eating correctly while losing weight, you may finally "burn off" body fat you already have stored *and* keep your energy levels high for months.

Some of the specific benefits of increased energy levels are as follows:

◆ Say good-bye to late-afternoon energy slumps. Those have been caused by blood sugar and insulin level swings. Your blood-sugar levels will become more stable throughout the day.

◆ You'll notice an increase in mental alertness. You'll have a steady supply of energy going to your brain from the energy supplied by fat burning, whereas energy from uneven blood sugar levels can contribute to *brain fog*.

◆ As insulin resistance abates, your body's cells can uptake more energy in the form of glucose. If you've had periods of fatigue in the past caused by insulin resistance, expect them to diminish.

> **Glyco Lingo**
>
> **Brain fog** is an unscientific term that describes the condition in which a person has difficulty thinking or behaving coherently. At those times a person could misplace keys—or children—and forget to do everyday chores. The person feels as if his or her IQ has dropped. This is often caused by low blood sugar levels, but it can also be caused by other more serious health conditions.

When you have more energy, you naturally participate in more activities. This contributes to further weight loss and starts a very positive upward spiral for weight-loss and lifestyle success.

Eating Patterns

If you've been on a restricted-calorie diet before, you know how hard it is to avoid overeating when you feel hungry all the time. Throw in the sudden and unexpected food cravings that can make a mess of your best intentions, and it's easy to see why staying on a restricted-calorie diet is agonizingly difficult and certainly not fun. On a glycemic index weight-loss program, however, it's easier to avoid both overeating and the challenging, and at times irresistible, food cravings. That kind of craving is produced by the restrictive nature of those diets.

Natural hunger—the kind you experience when your body actually needs food—is good because it signals that it's time to eat. But your natural hunger feelings can easily get confused with false hunger. False hunger comes when you feel compelled to eat more food than your body requires.

False hunger is often the result of swings in insulin levels. When you eat a high-carbohydrate meal or snack, your blood sugar is elevated and you feel satiated. Soon after that, however, your insulin levels increase quickly and lower your blood sugar levels. You feel hungry again. If you respond to this feeling by eating yet more high-glycemic, high-carb foods, you end up in an unsatisfying and fattening cycle. By eating mostly low-glycemic carbohydrates, you eliminate false hunger.

Food cravings are often a result of the same high-carb insulin-hunger cycle. You crave high-carb foods because they quickly increase your blood sugar levels and make you comfortable. Yes, it's usually carbs we crave. Very few of us—if anyone—who's caught up in an insulin-hunger cycle craves a fish fillet or a plain tossed salad. Instead, our cravings range from donuts and cookies to candy and bagels—foods that will keep the insulin-hunger cycle going strong. By avoiding the high-glycemic foods altogether, you avoid cravings and the insulin-hunger cycle.

Food cravings are also caused by stress. When times get tough and schedules become hectic, levels of the stress hormone cortisol rise. That's when many of us seek comfort foods such as mashed potatoes, rice pudding, and oatmeal cookies. These are among the foods that seem to lift our moods and soothe our stress, at least temporarily. But why?

These high-glycemic foods increase levels of the brain neurotransmitter *serotonin*. Serotonin soothes the brain and makes us feel relaxed. But—you guessed it—there's a downside. These foods make us fat, only work temporarily, and can ultimately increase anxiety and depression.

Glyco Lingo _____

Serotonin is a brain neurotransmitter responsible for relaxation and uplifted moods.

Here's how. These foods put us back on the insulin-hunger cycle in which our blood sugar is elevated but then crashes to a greater degree as excess insulin is delivered to the bloodstream. With lower-glycemic food intake, our insulin level is more stable.

Insulin and cortisol increase or decrease in tandem; so when people are stressed, their insulin and cortisol levels increase, which causes their body to store fat more readily. Ultimately, they gain weight. As insulin increases, so does cortisol. Cortisol uses up serotonin, which results in yet more feelings of anxiety, stress, and depression.

You'll learn more about how to manage your stress without eating high-glycemic carbohydrates in Chapter 23. But for now, know that you have plenty of excellent alternatives for lowering stress, ranging from meditation to exercise. Even sleep will restore serotonin levels.

$\textsf{THIN}$ **-couragement**

If you are suffering from serious mood disorders, such as depression, anxiety, or bipolar conditions, ask your health practitioner whether avoiding high-glycemic, high-carb foods could improve your situation. Many psychiatrists and psychologists now recommend avoiding most high-glycemic starches and other high-glycemic carbohydrates as part of an overall mental health regimen.

Mood Management

Eating high-glycemic food creates mood disorders. Your body reacts to these foods by increasing insulin levels, which then increases the level of stress hormones.

With elevated levels of adrenaline and cortisol, a person easily experiences anxiety, panic attacks, and depression. If stress hormones stay high over a long period of time, a person can end up medically diagnosed with a mood disorder.

As you control insulin levels with a glycemic index weight-loss program, you should feel better and have fewer down or anxious moments. This is a great win-win situation for someone trying to lose weight because just being on a weight-loss program often adds stress. So expect to feel good and feel in control of your moods, which makes for great weight-loss success.

Body Perks

Glycemic index weight loss offers you some terrific physical body benefits that you'll appreciate throughout your weight-loss program, including your maintenance program. Because we each have unique body chemistry and needs, the following benefits will vary:

◆ **Better and sounder sleep.** Because your stress levels won't be increased due to increased insulin and cortisol, more serotonin will be available, enabling you to get to sleep easier and to sleep more soundly. However, if your stress levels are already high because of other life situations, you might not fully realize this benefit.

◆ **Flatter tummy.** Yes, it takes plenty of exercise, crunches, sweat, and stretching to produce abs of steel. But if insulin and cortisol are raging through your body because of the insulin resistance, your ab crunching efforts won't produce the results you want. As your insulin levels stabilize at a lower level, you can expect to see a marked reduction in tummy flab. You can accelerate this result with an exercise program, as described in Part 6.

◆ **Regularity.** Because you'll be eating 25 grams or more of dietary fiber every day, you'll increase the transit time of food and remove waste products faster through your digestive system.

◆ **Fewer plateaus.** Weight-loss plateaus are the bane of people who are on any weight-loss program. You start losing weight but then plateau or level out, and no matter how rock-steady you are on your diet, you can't seem to lose the next few pounds. The stall seems unfair and can be so disappointing that a person loses momentum and enthusiasm. We can't promise that you won't experience a weight-loss plateau on a glycemic index weight-loss program, but provided you follow the total program of eating, exercise, and lifestyle changes, it will be short-lived and perhaps nonexistent.

◆ **Clearer skin.** Who doesn't want to have better skin? Elevated insulin levels cause inflammation, and the inflammation shows up in many areas of your body. One of them is your skin. Dermatologists now recommend a low-glycemic eating plan along with supplementation of omega-3 essential fatty acids to improve the appearance of your skin and make it moist, plump, and radiant. Eating right can reduce wrinkling, acne, breakouts, congestion, and other annoying skin conditions. You learn more about essential fatty acids in Chapter 12.

◆ **Fewer allergic reactions.** Research shows that people who eat meals based on the glycemic index tend to have fewer allergies or display milder symptoms. This is because lower insulin levels may enhance immune system function. Is it possible that you'll have fewer colds? We can't promise you, but it's possible.

◆ **Aging.** An important contributor to longevity is *insulin sensitivity*. Insulin sensitivity means your cells are responding to insulin and correctly taking up blood sugar for energy. By keeping your insulin levels low, the odds are you'll age better and live longer, too.

Glyco Lingo

Insulin sensitivity is a term that indicates the body's cells respond to insulin correctly. This is the opposite of insulin resistance, in which the body's cells don't respond adequately to insulin and therefore don't absorb nutrients, such as blood sugar, efficiently.

Of course, the biggest body perk is that you'll attain your ideal size and be able to stay there for life, simply by continuing to eat mostly low-glycemic foods and meals within the framework of a healthy lifestyle. No matter why you want to lose weight—to look good, for self-esteem, to move on with your life, or to improve your health—you'll have the opportunity to achieve your goals.

Health Benefits

By eating based on the glycemic index, you reduce your risk of ...

- Type 2 diabetes.

- Heart disease.

- High cholesterol, high triglycerides, lowered HDL, elevated LDL.

- High blood pressure.

- Autoimmune disease conditions, such as arthritis, allergies, fibromyalgia, and multiple sclerosis.

- Depression and anxiety.

- Alzheimer's and other dementias.

- Some cancers, including breast, colon, rectal, and endometrial cancers.

Research continues on the health benefits of eating based on the glycemic index. In the next few years, expect to read even more about why managing your insulin levels is advantageous to your health.

Appearance Benefits

Health and weight-loss benefits aren't all you can expect from eating the glycemic index way. Your appearance will benefit, too. Here are some of the possibilities:

- Better skin, nails, and hair

- Flatter tummy and midriff

- Fewer facial wrinkles

- Better muscle tone

- Less bloating

- More energy

- Uplifted moods

Now, what other diet program can come close to offering all or some of the above? These benefits come from better nutrition, from avoiding starvation metabolism, and from reducing inflammation.

Feeding the Whole Family

After you learn how to locate, prepare, and eat low-glycemic foods, you'll be delighted with how easy it is. You'll also be amazed at how good the foods taste. You'll learn how to eat in virtually any restaurant and how to prepare meals quickly and simply. We give you plenty of meal ideas later in this book, and you can also use the recipes in *The Complete Idiot's Guide Glycemic Index Cookbook*, *The Complete Idiot's Guide to Low-Carb Meals*, and *The Complete Idiot's Guide to Terrific Diabetic Meals* as guides for eating.

With some modifications, your glycemic index weight-loss program can work well for every member of your family. Remember, not only can individuals lose weight by eating mostly low-glycemic foods, they also gain marvelous health benefits. Certainly you want those health benefits for everyone in your family and for all your friends. You can serve low-glycemic foods at parties, take low-glycemic prepared dishes to potluck dinners, and feed your family and friends every day with the same foods you'll be eating on a glycemic index weight-loss plan.

Not limiting food choices and not counting calories are terrific benefits to being on a glycemic index weight-loss program. On past diets, you may have sat at dinner night after night watching your teenage children and spouse devour pizzas or burgers while you ate a slice of Melba toast, some dry chicken breast, and a small green salad dressed with lemon juice. Those days are over.

It's much more fun to fit in socially when you eat with others and not draw attention to yourself and your food needs. Now you won't have to. You'll need to learn a few "tricks" and techniques—which come later in the book—but you don't have to feel like the odd person out at any meal.

The Least You Need to Know

- ◆ Your energy levels will be higher and more balanced when you are eating the low-glycemic index way.

- ◆ You avoid the intense hunger and food cravings of other types of dieting when eating low-glycemic foods.

- ◆ Glycemic index weight-loss programs help you reduce stress, improve sleep, and minimize dieting plateaus.

- ◆ Your overall health and appearance will improve with a glycemic index weight-loss program.

4

What Makes a Carbohydrate Low Glycemic

In This Chapter

- Learning glycemic index food facts
- Comparing high-glycemic and low-glycemic carbs
- Identifying digestible carbs
- Understanding processed and unprocessed carbohydrates

The world of carbohydrates comes with its own vocabulary. You've heard such terms as complex carbohydrates and refined sugars. Plus, you've probably heard about "bad carbs" and "good carbs," as if carbs are either angelic or demonic. The terms have become part of our collective weight-loss jargon.

Don't worry. There's no reason why the glycemic index has to be weighty, vague, or confusing. You won't need expert knowledge to know which carbohydrates you should eat and which ones to eat sparingly. We simplify the terminology and make it easy to understand.

It's highly useful for you to have a fundamental understanding of the glycemic index. The knowledge will help you make wise food choices in your daily life. In this chapter, you learn about the different categories of carbohydrates, and you learn more about how they relate to the glycemic index.

Some Simple Rules of Thumb

As this chapter explains the differences between carbohydrates, keep in mind the following guidelines. Think of them as "rules of thumb" that you need to modify to your personal weight-loss needs:

◆ Highly refined carbohydrates are usually high glycemic. These include the classic "white" flour and also any whole grain that's finely milled, such as whole wheat flour. "Popped" grains and cereals such as popcorn and rice cakes are also high glycemic. So are white potatoes.

◆ White sugar is medium glycemic, whereas the glycemic index of honey varies based on origin. Single-flower honeys are usually low glycemic, while those from a mixture of flowers are usually medium glycemic.

◆ The slower a complex carb breaks down into its simple sugars in your digestive tract, the lower glycemic it is. Stone-ground wheat bread takes more time to digest in your stomach than whole wheat or white bread, so its glycemic index is lower.

◆ Dietary fiber slows down starch and sugar absorption in the stomach, and so consequently lowers the glycemic index.

Body of Knowledge

Dietary fiber that's actually part of the food, as in brown rice or stone-ground flour, is usually better for lowering the glycemic index of a food rather than adding fiber, such as oat or wheat bran, to refined, finely milled flour. However, if a large portion, ⅓ to ½ of the total dry ingredients, is unprocessed wheat bran, oat bran, or psyllium, the glycemic index can end up being low. For low-glycemic bread recipes see *The Complete Idiot's Guide to Terrific Diabetic Meals.*

◆ Naturally occurring unprocessed carbohydrates, such as vegetables, whole kernel grains, and fruits, are lower glycemic than processed carbohydrates, such as baked goods and candy.

◆ Nutrient-dense carbohydrates are healthier for you because they contain more important vitamins, minerals, antioxidants, and other micronutrients. These are usually the unprocessed and un-prepackaged foods.

◆ Rice that's low glycemic is basmati rice and Uncle Ben's converted rice. The glycemic index of other rice varieties may be high or medium.

◆ Resistant starch is generally lower in glycemic value and higher in healthy fiber than nonresistant starches. You can make certain starches resistant by cooking, then chilling and eating cold or at room temperature. Starches that qualify are white potatoes, corn, rice, barley, legumes, and bananas.

As you eat based on the glycemic index, you'll gain an instinctive knowledge about which foods will trigger a rise in your blood sugar levels and which ones won't. Until then, plan your meals with a glycemic index list close at hand.

Body of Knowledge

It's possible that some low-glycemic or medium-glycemic foods react in your body as if they were high glycemic. Researchers don't know why this happens, but it does. If you suspect a food works differently for you, by all means, eat it carefully. For example, bananas may seem high glycemic to you, but actually, they're listed as low glycemic at 52.

Easy or Hard to Digest

The faster your body can digest a carbohydrate, the higher its glycemic index value. There are two major types of digestible polysaccharides or complex carbohydrates: amylose and amylopectin. Both contain many glucose units, but the foods with more amylopectin raise the blood glucose levels much more readily than foods containing more amylose. The branches in amylopectin starch have many surface areas, which make it easier for digestive enzymes to break it down faster.

These easy-to-break-down starches include foods such as most breads, white potatoes, white flour, and snack foods such as pretzels, donuts, and cookies. Most of these foods contain processed or refined carbohydrates, but some natural unprocessed carbohydrates have higher amylopectin levels, including parsnips, russet potatoes, and rutabagas.

Starches that contain more amylose include some whole grains and legumes (lentils, dried peas, and beans) and some of the starchy vegetables such as yams and sweet potatoes. These foods are best for your glycemic index weight-loss program.

The exception is resistant starches, which are created in white potatoes, rice, corn, barley, legumes, and bananas when cooked, chilled, and then eaten cold or at room temperature.

Dietary Fiber

Most dietary fiber is not digestible. In other words, you might consume the fiber as you eat fiber-containing foods. It passes through the digestive system and is excreted in your stool. Fiber adds bulk and slows the stomach's absorption of starches and sugars. Fiber helps lower the glycemic effect of a meal. It's good to eat lots of fiber—from 25 to 45 grams per day.

Don't overdo the fiber. But you'd need to consume a virtually unpalatable amount of fiber supplements, such as psyllium husks, to eat too much fiber—such as 4 or 5 tablespoons a day. With too much fiber, you could actually block the absorption of important vitamins, minerals, amino acids, and more. Overeating fiber can, in essence, make you undernourished. (And undernourished doesn't equate to being thinner.) More than 45 grams of fiber a day is generally too much. You can find fiber counts for carbohydrates in Appendix B.

Refined and Unrefined Carbohydrates

Another distinction that some nutritional counselors make is between refined and unrefined carbohydrates. In glycemic index weight loss, we prefer to classify carbohydrates as low, medium, or high glycemic. However, because you're bound to hear carbohydrates defined as refined and unrefined, this section discusses how the terminology relates to the glycemic index.

Refined carbohydrates are more highly processed than unrefined carbohydrates. Processing includes such activities as cooking, milling, and separating the whole food into parts. Examples of refined carbohydrates are fluffy whole wheat bread, white bread, white rice, most packaged breakfast cereals, donuts, cakes, cookies, bagels, fruit and vegetable juices, fruit drinks, soda, and candy. Refined carbs are usually high glycemic, but some can be low, as in vegetable juice and some fruit juices.

Unrefined carbohydrates are those sold and eaten in their natural state. In general, unrefined carbohydrates tend to contain more fiber. Examples of unrefined carbohydrates are whole vegetables and fruit, whole grains, dried peas and beans, and nuts and seeds. Some foods are processed more than others. For example, fruit juice is not processed as much as fruit drinks. Usually unrefined carbs are low glycemic, but not always, so be sure to check the glycemic index listings before you eat them.

Pastas

Even though regular pasta is a highly refined, processed carbohydrate, its glycemic value can be low, medium, or high, depending on how you cook it. If you cook spaghetti for only 5 to 6 minutes, just until it's barely al dente, it's low glycemic. Other types of pasta may need slightly more or less cooking time. If you open a can of prepared spaghetti in sauce, those noodles will have a high glycemic index because they're mushy.

Cook pasta just until it softens and you'll be eating a healthier meal. The longer pasta is cooked, the more available the starch is for quick digestion—exactly what you don't want. If the pasta sticks on the wall when you test for doneness, it's overcooked. Don't eat mushy pasta.

The Good, the Bad, and the Glycemic Index

Carbohydrates aren't good or bad; the difference is in how you eat them and how much of them you eat. This is one of the reasons why glycemic index weight loss works so well. You don't need to give up your favorite treat food, whether white bread, bagels, or candy bars. But you do need to eat them in such a way that you don't cause a quick rise in your blood sugar levels, and you must watch portion sizes.

The glycemic index gives you a way of managing your blood sugar and insulin levels, thus assuring that you aren't storing fat and also that you continue to lose weight.

One way to do this is to manage your glycemic load by meal and by day. You'll be balancing the low-glycemic foods with some high and some medium, and overall, you can keep your insulin levels low. For example, it's better to have a small piece of high-glycemic dessert after a balanced dinner of meat and vegetables than it is to eat that same small piece of dessert midafternoon all by itself. You'll learn more about the glycemic load in Chapter 5.

THIN-couragement

Angela loved eating sugar. In fact, she'd never met a sweet treat that she didn't want to eat. Her intense sugar cravings bothered her and she wanted to lose about 30 pounds. She embarked on a glycemic index weight-loss program and decided that it was very easy for her to give up breads and wheat products to eat mostly low glycemic. But she didn't want to stop all sugary foods. And she didn't need to. In her food plan, she was able to savor two ounces of dark chocolate twice a week, and still lose weight.

Now's the time to give up the notion of bad and good carbs and of fattening and non-fattening carbs and to accept all carbs as okay, based on how you eat them.

The Acid Factor

The only way to describe how acidic foods affect the glycemic index is to say it's un-expected. Who would have thought that eating an acidic-tasting or sour-tasting food with a carbohydrate would lower the effective glycemic index? Most likely, no one.

Yet that's exactly what happens. Acidic foods significantly lower the glycemic index of a food or a meal by as much as one third. The reason lies in how your stomach and digestive system work. Acidic foods slow the emptying of your stomach. The acidic foods slow down your digestion, which slows down how quickly your blood sugar rises.

Yes this is a wonderful boon to your weight-loss program. You can manage the glycemic effect of your meals by what you eat. Here's a list of foods that are acidic:

- Cocoa that's not Dutch processed
- Coffee, black
- Chutney
- Dill and sweet pickles
- Grapefruit, lemons, limes, and green teas
- Green olives
- Horseradish
- Kumquats
- Lemon juice
- Lime juice
- Marinated vegetables, such as artichokes, mushrooms, carrots, and green beans

- Pickled beets
- Pickled eggs
- Pickled garlic
- Pickled herring
- Pickled legumes
- Pickled peppers, such as jalapeños
- Sauerbraten
- Sauerkraut
- Sourdough bread
- Tangy salsas
- Vinegar
- Vinegar-and-oil salad dressings

THIN -couragement _____

> If you love croutons on your salads, but don't want to eat high-glycemic breads, make your own croutons with sourdough bread. Cut the bread into small cubes and lightly sauté in olive oil or butter and spices, such as Italian seasoning. Store them in an airtight bag in the refrigerator. Use just a few—they add great flavor and crunch.

Some of the acidic foods, such as pickled beets, chutney, some of the marinated vegetables, and sweet pickles, have added sugar. Consequently, we don't recommend eating them in large quantity—the glycemic load would be too high.

THIN -couragement _____

> In using the glycemic index for weight loss, Sally learned that her body simply couldn't handle white bread. Within minutes of eating it, she would feel bloated and uncomfortable. By the next day, her clothes were tighter. This was the case with all bread except for sourdough bread. She can eat a small piece of sourdough bread once or twice a week with a complete meal without any side effects or weight gain. The difference is that sourdough bread is acidic. And the more sour, the better for weight loss.

Use the acidic foods as condiments and side dishes to your meals and snacks. Toss your salads with vinegar-and-oil salad dressings. You need four teaspoons of vinegar on your salad to reduce the glycemic value of your meal by about 30 percent. Use lemon to flavor your herbal teas and your water at meals. Make guacamole salad with fresh-squeezed lime juice.

Think of a balanced meal as containing animal protein, vegetables, and an acidic food. Your waistline will be glad you do.

Don't Count These Carbs

Some carbohydrates aren't listed in the glycemic index. They simply don't contain enough carbohydrate to affect your blood sugar levels. These are most of the non-starchy vegetables. On average these vegetables contain about 5 grams of carbohydrates for 1 cup raw or ½ cup cooked vegetables. Lettuce varieties, including raw spinach, contain about two grams of carbohydrates per one cup raw lettuce—so for salad greens, use it as a free food.

Body of Knowledge _____

The spice, cinnamon, has been shown to lower blood glucose levels in persons with diabetes. Here's how to use cinnamon for weight loss. If you add cinnamon as a flavoring to foods, such as sweet potatoes or herbal teas, you could effectively lower the glycemic effect of a meal. But use only small quantities, between ¼ to 1 teaspoon a day. Don't use larger amounts because one of the flavorings in cinnamon, coumarin, can cause mutations or cancer if eaten in large amounts. The toxic components in cinnamon are insoluble, so if you want to consume more than what's indicated here, boil the cinnamon in water and pour off the soluble part for use and then discard the solid part.

Here's a list of foods you can eat freely without concern to glycemic index or load:

- Alfalfa sprouts
- Artichokes
- Asparagus
- Bamboo shoots
- Broccoli
- Cabbage
- Carrots, raw
- Cauliflower
- Celery
- Celery root
- Chard, Swiss
- Collards
- Cucumber
- Eggplant
- Endive
- Fennel
- Green beans
- Hearts of palm
- Jicama
- Kale
- Lettuce
- Mushrooms
- Mustard greens
- Okra
- Onions
- Parsley
- Pea pods
- Peppers (both bell and chili)
- Radicchio
- Radishes
- Sauerkraut
- Scallions
- Spinach
- Squash, summer

- ◆ Squash, zucchini
- ◆ Tomatillos
- ◆ Tomatoes
- ◆ Turnip greens

- ◆ Turnips
- ◆ Water chestnuts
- ◆ Watercress

Other foods not classified as nonstarchy veggies, but also very low in carbohydrates and with a "0" glycemic index, include the following:

- ◆ Avocados contain good monounsaturated fat, which can lower cholesterol levels.

- ◆ Chayote is a fruit, is high in nutrients, has no fat, and contains only 5 grams of carbs per cup. It has a 0 glycemic index value.

- ◆ Nuts and seeds are a natural food that contains good fat and vegetable protein. They have a low to a 0 glycemic index value and 1 or less glycemic load per serving. Peanuts (actually a legume) and cashews contain a small amount of carbohydrates, but they're both low glycemic.

So go ahead and eat these healthful vegetables and nuts. In the quantities recommended, they're packed with valuable nutrition, they don't raise your blood sugar levels, and they don't stimulate insulin overproduction.

Yes, your mother was right: you should eat your vegetables … especially these!

The Least You Need to Know

- ◆ Carbohydrates can be fattening or thinning, based on how you eat them. The more slowly a carbohydrate is digested, the lower its glycemic index.

- ◆ Eating high-fiber foods with a meal lowers the glycemic value of the entire meal.

- ◆ Pasta can be low, medium, or high glycemic, based on how long you cook it.

- ◆ Processed foods generally have a higher glycemic value than their unprocessed counterparts.

- ◆ Eating acidic-tasting foods with a meal can lower the glycemic effect by as much as 30 percent.

- ◆ Some carbs, such as the nonstarchy vegetables that contain a very small quantity of carbs, have a glycemic index of 0, so they don't have any impact on your glycemic load.

Chapter 5

Tallying Your Glycemic Load

In This Chapter

◆ Balancing quality with glycemic value

◆ Calculating glycemic load

◆ Eating acidic foods

◆ Determining the glycemic load for a recipe or a meal

One thing's for certain. Our bodies and how they process food are very complex. The old-time formula for weight loss, "eat less and exercise more," is just too simplistic.

The glycemic index is based on the complex, interrelated aspects of how our bodies process what we eat. Unfortunately, at first the glycemic index can seem complex, too. But don't be intimidated by it. It's fundamentally simple. And as you learn more, you'll appreciate how brilliantly it aligns with how your body's digestion and metabolism functions.

So let's explore the glycemic index a little deeper. In this chapter you learn how the amount of low-, medium- or high-glycemic carbohydrates you eat makes a difference in your weight-loss results. You've already learned about the quality of carbohydrates, now we'll discuss amounts of food by calculating the glycemic load.

Wrong Weigh

Because low-glycemic foods aid in hunger satisfaction, it is harder to overeat with low-glycemic carbohydrate foods, but not impossible. Eating too many low-glycemic carbohydrates can increase your overall glycemic load and slow or even halt your weight loss. Be sure you take into account the amount you eat as well as the quality, to achieve your desired weight-loss goals.

Quantity and Quality

The glycemic load is the key to knowing how much of a carb to eat. As you have already learned, the glycemic index gives you information about the quality of a carbohydrate. The numerical value tells you how eating that carbohydrate will affect your blood sugar levels. The glycemic index alone, however, doesn't give you a guide for how much of any carbohydrate you can or should eat.

When the glycemic index first became popular, many people assumed that as long as a food was low glycemic, it didn't matter how much of it they ate. Wrong. Indiscriminately filling up on too many carbohydrates, even low-glycemic ones, causes weight gain.

Yes, quantity makes a big difference, which means we need a simple way to calculate how to eat "glycemically smart" throughout the day. That's where the glycemic load comes in handy. It's a more precise guide of how many carbohydrates to eat *and* how to eat a balanced low-glycemic diet.

Calculating Glycemic Load

Even though you won't need a pencil, paper, and calculator to compute the glycemic load of your meals, it's helpful to understand how glycemic load is calculated.

Body of Knowledge

New glycemic index tables include the glycemic load for average serving sizes. Until recently, the tables were calculated for countries such as Canada and Australia that measure food quantities in grams. This made it challenging for us in the United States to use glycemic load. Most of us don't know how to convert grams into ounces and then into cups and tablespoons. Fortunately, the glycemic index has become so popular that newer glycemic charts give quantities in more familiar measurements such as cups and ounces.

To calculate the glycemic load of a quantity of a carbohydrate, multiply the glycemic index value times the quantity of carbohydrates of the serving in grams, then divide by 100. The equation looks like this:

GI value × grams of carbohydrates per serving ÷ 100 = glycemic load

Here's an example of the difference in glycemic load between a five-ounce serving of baked white potato and a five-ounce serving of baked yams:

Baked white potatoes:

5 ounces

34 grams carbohydrates

Glycemic index is 85 (high glycemic)

Glycemic load is 29 or (34 × 85) ÷ 100

Baked yams:

5 ounces

34 grams carbohydrates

Glycemic index is 37 (low glycemic)

Glycemic load is 13 or (34 × 37) ÷100

The glycemic load of white potatoes is twice that of the yams, so its effect on a person's blood sugar is twice as great as eating the yams. This is a very significant difference in terms of weight loss. Remember, you want to keep your insulin levels low and this is how you do it—by eating a low-glycemic load.

THIN-couragement

At a large family dinner, Lucy baked an equal amount of white potatoes and yams and put both in a bowl on the dinner table. She wanted to observe which ones her teenage sons and their friends would eat. She didn't mention the nutritional or glycemic index value; in fact, she didn't say anything about them at all. As she cleared the table, she observed that all the yams had been eaten while plenty of white baked potatoes remained. Seems the teens thought the baked yams were more appetizing. Most likely, you will, too.

Let's look at another example, this time with dessert.

Tofu-based frozen dessert, chocolate, sweetened with high-fructose corn syrup:

> ½ cup
>
> 30 grams carbohydrate
>
> Glycemic index is 115
>
> Glycemic load is 34

Premium ice cream:

> ½ cup
>
> 15 carbohydrate grams
>
> Glycemic index is 37
>
> Glycemic load is 5

Yes, a half cup of absolutely rich and luscious premium ice cream has a glycemic load of only 5. The supposedly "healthy" tofu-based frozen dessert has a load of 34.

So which is healthier for your heart, your insulin levels, insulin resistance, and more? The correct answer is the premium ice cream, provided that you eat no more than ½ cup and the amount of saturated fat is within your limits for that day. Isn't this great? If ice cream is not a *trigger food* for you, you can have some ice cream and lose weight, too.

> **Glyco Lingo** _____
>
> A **trigger food** is one that can lead you to overeating—or even to binge eating. Some common trigger foods are candy, chips, popcorn, donuts, and ice cream. If you have a trigger food and find it impossible to eat only a small amount, it's best not to eat it at all.

High, Medium, and Low Loads

By now you're familiar with how individual carbohydrates are classified based on their glycemic index value: high, 70 and over; medium, 56 to 69; and low, 55 or lower.

Now we need to introduce you to how carbohydrate portions are categorized based on the glycemic load.

A glycemic load of 20 or above is high, 11 to 19 is medium, and 10 or below is low. The serving of yams in the previous example is medium while the serving of white potatoes is high. The glycemic load of the tofu frozen dessert is high and the ice cream is low.

As a review, to calculate glycemic load (GL), both the grams of carbohydrates and the glycemic index are put into the calculation. GL equals carbohydrate grams times glycemic index divided by 100. If a very small amount of a high-glycemic food is eaten, it does not have a big impact. However, research indicates that the more frequently you eat high-glycemic foods, such as the tofu frozen dessert, the more likely you are to experience weight gain and health risks. The reason for this appears to be that the higher-glycemic foods do not satisfy hunger as well as the low-glycemic foods do. So in practice, it's better to eat mostly low-glycemic foods and only eat high-glycemic items sparingly, if at all. In this comparison, you'd be better off choosing the ice cream. Your waistline will celebrate—or at least be smaller.

Body of Knowledge

If you don't want to calculate the glycemic load, you can count carbs. To start, allow 30 grams of low-glycemic carbohydrates per meal and 10 to 30 grams of low-glycemic carbohydrates for snacks. Eat three meals and two to three snacks. Eat only low-glycemic carbohydrates. Count all carbohydrates, even the nonstarchy "free food" vegetables. The total grams of carbohydrates for the entire day with meals and snacks should be less than 150. Some people may need to keep their carb total between 90 to 120 to lose weight.

Your Daily Allotment

The key to success with glycemic index weight loss is simple: eat within your glycemic load allotment every day. Here are some guidelines for choosing your allotment. Start with these recommendations and then modify them if necessary. You may need to lower them if you aren't losing weight, or raise them if you are losing too quickly.

◆ Start with a glycemic load allotment of 60 to 75 per day, making sure to spread this out over the course of the day. You might have 15 at each meal and three snacks of about 10 each.

◆ If you are pregnant or nursing, you'll need to increase your glycemic load to as much as 130 per day. It is not recommended to diet while you are pregnant or in the first four months of nursing.

- A highly active woman or man may need to eat a glycemic load of between 100 to 150 to give them plenty of energy. Men usually need to eat a higher glycemic load because they weigh more than women and have more muscle mass.

- A younger person needs to eat a higher glycemic load than a person who is older, because metabolism slows with age.

- A person with a lower percentage of body fat can eat a higher daily allotment than a person with a high body fat percentage because he or she has a higher metabolism.

Start with the previous recommendations. After several weeks, you'll learn how the different carbohydrates work in your body. And if you aren't losing weight, lower your glycemic load allotment to 50 to 60 until you are losing weight and your clothes fit looser. It is not healthy for most of us to go lower than a 50 glycemic load.

Wrong Weigh _____

Janice found what she thought was a great way to get her five servings of vegetables and fruits every day. For lunch, she made a smoothie of a banana, a cup of fruit juice, strawberries, cherries, and pineapple. She added some yogurt and ice and voilà! She was obtaining all her necessary antioxidants, vitamins, and fiber in one single meal. Plus, she didn't need to mess with any more vegetables or fruit the rest of the day. Whoa. Just a minute. The glycemic load of that smoothie was off the charts. Not only that, somehow she missed the vegetable part of the government's recommendations. No wonder she wasn't losing weight but, rather, gaining it.

Another lesson here is that you shouldn't "save up" your glycemic load allotment and eat it all at one meal. You won't be able to lose weight if you do. Instead, you'll be triggering your body's fat-storing system with a rapid increase in blood sugar and insulin levels.

Combination Foods

The glycemic index and the glycemic load work very well for individual foods. So far, so good. But what if you want to fix your favorite recipe? How can you figure out the glycemic index or the glycemic load?

In a scientific sense, you can't calculate the glycemic index of a combination of ingredients. The very fact of the combination changes the value. For example, pizza is a very complex food. The crust is made of white or whole-wheat bread, which would make it high glycemic. The tomato sauce is medium glycemic. The meats and cheeses in the topping are zero, as they contain virtually no carbs but they do contain fat. If you intuitively average the glycemic indexes, you'd guess that pizza is medium glycemic. But, actually, pizza is low glycemic with a glycemic load of about nine per slice.

Let's look at the factors that contribute to this surprising result:

- The starch, in this case the flour, is enriched and in very fine particles, so the starch is easily digested, making it high glycemic.

- Pizza is low in fiber, which would make it a high-glycemic food.

- Pizza is a high-fat food. Fat slows down digestion, so the starch isn't as quickly digested as if the bread were eaten alone.

- Tomatoes are acidic, as are some of the possible toppings, such as olives, peppers, and pepperoni. Acid slows down the digestion of starch.

Now, here's the problem. Although pizza is a low-glycemic food, beware. Eat it sparingly, if at all. Here's why. Pizza bread is high glycemic and you don't want to overdo high-glycemic foods, even if they are balanced with acid and fat. Plus, it's important to keep your saturated fat at about 10 percent of your daily food intake, which is really hard to do when you eat more than one piece of pizza. So one slice of pizza now and then—say once a week—is fine. Be sure to add a fresh green salad with vinegar-and-oil dressing to add fiber and an acid food to the meal.

One of the big weight-loss challenges with foods such as pizza, cookies, and donuts is that it's hard to stop with just one. Even though some could be low or medium glycemic because they contain eggs and fat, they can still ruin your weight-loss efforts if you eat more than a small amount. Eat only one slice of pizza or one cookie or even just a half so that you gain taste satisfaction but not pounds. Or better yet, in the case of pizza, eat the topping and hold the crust. Overeating is always fattening—it increases insulin resistance all by itself.

Calculations for Meals and Recipes

You can calculate the glycemic index and glycemic load for recipes and meals. Joan did this for every recipe in our cookbooks *The Complete Idiot's Guide Glycemic Index Cookbook* and *The Complete Idiot's Guide to Terrific Diabetic Meals*. However, we don't recommend you do these calculations on a day-to-day basis unless you love arithmetic, calculators, doing ratios, and other aspects of mathematics.

Here's how to calculate the glycemic index of a recipe. The result of your calculation will be an estimate only. The only way to know the exact glycemic index is to test it on volunteers in a research setting. But we find an estimate to be just fine for everyday eating.

Step 1: List all carbohydrate ingredients and the amount of carbohydrates for each ingredient. You can find this for most carbohydrates in Appendix B. List all ingredients whether or not they contain carbohydrates.

Step 2: Add the total of carbohydrates to determine how many carbs are in the recipe or meal.

Step 3: By doing ratios, determine what percentage of the total carbs comes from each ingredient.

Step 4: Multiply the percentage of each ingredient by its glycemic index value.

Step 5: Add all the values from step 4 together. This is the calculated glycemic index of the recipe or meal.

Here's how to calculate the glycemic load of a serving for a meal or recipe.

Step 1: Start with the calculated glycemic index of the recipes or meals from step 5.

Step 2: Multiply by the total number of grams of carbohydrates in the recipe or meal.

Step 3: Divide the number in step 2 by the number of servings in the recipe.

Step 4: Divide the number by 100. That's the glycemic load.

Body of Knowledge

Doing the calculations for the glycemic load of combination foods, such as recipes and meals, can't give you a truly accurate answer, but you can get close. The glycemic index of a food can vary based on where it's grown, how long it ripened, and the kind of soil in which it was grown. Also, when ingredients are cooked together, the glycemic index changes. But because eating isn't an exact science anyway, getting close can provide you with valuable and useful information.

Example:

Chicken Broccoli and Pasta with Slivered Almonds

Serves: 2

Serving size: 2 cups

Ingredients	Carb Grams	Percentage	Glycemic Index
Broccoli 2 cups	10	.22	0
Red pepper 1 cup	5	.11	0
Whole wheat pasta ⅔ cup	30	.66	32
Olive oil 1 tsp.	0	0	0
Chicken 6 oz.	0	0	0
Sliced almonds 2 TB.	2	.04	0
Totals	47	21 (.66 × 32 = 21)	

21 is the GI for the recipe. To calculate GL for this example, because it contains 2 servings, it is:

GI × carb/serving or 21 × 23 ÷ by 100 = 4.83 or 5.

5 × 21 ÷ 10 = 10.5

10.5 is the GL per serving. To determine the GL per serving:

For this recipe, 5 is the GL and 21 is the GI.

The above calculations don't account for some ingredients that could lower the effective glycemic index and glycemic load. Fats, proteins, and acids can change the result. As of now, there's no way to predict how much these kinds of ingredients would change your results. That's why the above is only an estimate.

Whew! If you're not into calculations, you may want an easier way to determine what and how much to eat. In Chapter 10, you'll find the Keep It Simple program that doesn't require any calculations.

Possible Discrepancies

The glycemic index is a scientific development and, as such, it's still in the process of being completely understood. There are some things we don't have complete theories for:

- How much the fats in a meal lower the effective glycemic index.
- Why cinnamon lowers the glycemic effect of a meal.

◆ How to predict the effect that protein has on blood sugar when eaten with a carbohydrate and fat.

◆ How much a high-stress life can change the effective glycemic index and glycemic load of a meal.

◆ If a carbohydrate of starch reacts in the body the same way a carbohydrate of fruit does. The underlying assumption in the glycemic index theory is that they react in the same way, but this is still not verified as scientifically correct.

◆ How to predict individual variations such as genetics, gender, age, health, and medications.

Stay tuned to learn more about the glycemic index as more information becomes available.

The Least You Need to Know

◆ The amount of carbohydrates you eat is measured by the glycemic load.

◆ Acid-based foods can lower the glycemic load of a meal by as much as one third.

◆ You can calculate the glycemic index and load of a recipe and a meal or use the charts and cookbook nutritional tables.

◆ Eat low-glycemic carbohydrates throughout the day, two to three per meal to avoid glycemic loading.

Part 2

Designing Your Glycemic Index Weight-Loss Program

You'll begin by learning how to keep your metabolism high and progress to choosing one of two glycemic index weight-loss programs, either the Keep It Simple or the Comprehensive program. You'll be able to stay the course using the power of your mind coupled with affirmations to visualize yourself at your ideal size.

Your maintenance program is the same as your weight-loss program, but you'll be eating more medium- and high-glycemic carbohydrates. As you attain your ideal size, you'll feel so good and have such high energy that you'll find yourself falling in love with this healthful way of eating.

Chapter 6

Keeping Your Metabolism High

In This Chapter

◆ Understanding metabolic resistance

◆ Boosting your metabolism

◆ Using low-glycemic eating to lift the basal metabolic rate

◆ Identifying causes of metabolism slowdown

Perhaps you've thought something like this as the pounds have crept on: "If only my metabolism were higher, I never would have gained all this weight in the first place. I would be able to eat whatever I wanted, whenever I wanted, and never gain a pound."

Unfortunately, this is magical thinking. Very few people can eat anything at any time and maintain a healthy weight for life. However, your metabolism is an important factor in your weight and ability to lose weight. Your basal metabolic rate plays a major role in your glycemic index weight-loss success.

Decreasing body fat and increasing muscle mass is only one method for increasing your basal metabolic rate. In this chapter, you learn more ways to increase your metabolism during your glycemic index weight-loss program. You'll also be able to identify your personal challenges to boosting your metabolism.

What's Slowing Your Metabolism?

Although some people can keep their metabolism high throughout their lives, most can't. Certain biological factors are, well, facts of life. After a person's biological prime, say at about age 30 or 35, the body's hormonal system begins to slow down and continues slowing down with every passing decade. As hormone production slows, so, too, does the *basal metabolic rate.*

With a slower metabolism, the body naturally increases fat storage while slowing down the production of muscle mass. As a person gains more body fat, metabolism slows down further, creating a cycle that keeps metabolism low and fat storage high. The reason your body does this is that it takes more energy, or calories, to maintain a pound of muscle than a pound of fat. So if we compare two women who are the same height, weight, and age, the woman who has a body fat percentage of 25 percent will typically have a higher metabolism than the woman who has a body fat percentage of 35 percent. Quite simply, lower body fat percentage translates into a higher metabolism. So one goal for increasing your metabolism is to increase your muscle mass and decrease your body fat percentage.

Glyco Lingo

Basal metabolic rate is the rate at which a person's body uses energy when relaxed or sedentary. The body really does "burn" through food, actually producing heat and providing energy to your organs and muscles. (Sometimes it is referred to as the thermic or thermogenic effect of your body.)

A diet high in carbohydrates—especially high-glycemic carbohydrates—increases insulin levels. Excess insulin stores excess blood sugar as fat. Too much insulin increases a person's body fat stores and body fat percentage, eventually slowing metabolism.

Fortunately, the opposite is also true. When you eat the low-glycemic way, your body produces less insulin. When insulin levels are low, your body isn't continuing to store fat. A low-glycemic weight-loss program makes your body use its own stored fat for energy, so your body fat percentage drops, your metabolism rises, and you lose weight! All this, plus, you'll find it easier to maintain your weight loss.

Metabolic Resistance

Some people have such slow metabolisms that losing weight is very difficult. These people have *metabolic resistance*. This is often caused by having too much body fat, but it can also be caused by other factors that include decreased mobility, genetic predisposition to insulin resistance, hormonal imbalances due to medications, poor sleep, a sedentary lifestyle, toxin buildup, severe dieting, and stress. Ideal body fat percentages are as follows:

Women:	Up to age 20	14–21%
	Ages 20 to 50	17–27%
	Age 50+	20–30%
Men:	Up to age 20	9–15%
	Ages 20 to 50	14–21%
	Age 50+	19–23%

Within these ranges, your metabolism is working at top performance and you won't look overweight. Use this chart to set your desired body fat percentage. You can have your current body fat percentage measured at a health club or fitness center. There are many ways to measure body fat, including bioimpedance, near-infrared interactance, dual-energy x-ray absorptiometry, underwater body measuring, MRI (magnetic resonance imaging), CT (computerized tomography), and body composition by air displacement. The important thing is to consistently use the same method on a regular basis. That way you'll get a more reliable measure of progress.

Glyco Lingo

Metabolic resistance is a condition in which a person's basal metabolic rate is so low that the person has a difficult time losing weight and increasing muscle.

A person can also become metabolically resistant to weight loss because of many years of yo-yo dieting, usually by limiting fat or calories. Yo-yo dieting encourages the body to increase fat storage because insulin levels can remain high during both the weight-loss times and the weight-gain times. Remember, not all diet programs keep insulin levels low. In fact, most don't; so a person could lose pounds and still gain fat.

Another factor that can contribute to metabolic resistance is leading a sedentary lifestyle. The sofa, the office chair, and screen time are your enemies! The more you move, the easier it is to lose weight. If you suspect that you're metabolically resistant to weight loss, be sure to add daily exercise, both strength training and aerobics, to your low-glycemic weight-loss program. Exercise lavishly and you'll banish metabolic resistance.

Boosting Your Metabolism

Nothing can be done about your age, so don't worry about it. You simply are the age you are, and yes, your metabolism slows down accordingly. Be sure you aren't using your age as an excuse for being overweight. You can rev up your metabolism in spite of your age. Here's what to do in addition to eating the low-glycemic way.

Avoid Overeating

Low-glycemic weight loss only works to the extent that you don't overeat. When you overeat, your body's insulin levels become elevated and your body starts storing fat.

When low-carb diets, as opposed to low-glycemic weight-loss programs, first became popular in the 1970s, many well-intentioned experts believed that individuals could eat as much fat and meat as they wanted, provided they avoided most carbohydrates, even vegetables and fruit.

What we know today, 20 years later, is that it's not healthy or a good idea to overeat any food, be it fat, protein, or carbohydrates. The good news is that it is much harder to overeat when eating low-glycemic carbohydrates. You will find eating low glycemic to be very satisfying and it will help with hunger satisfaction.

The size of your unstretched stomach is about the size of your fist. So make a fist right now and take a look at the volume we're talking about. Your body needs about that much food three or four times a day. If you eat much more than that at a sitting, you're overeating and slowing down your metabolism in the process.

A friend says it best this way: she hates the feeling of overeating and now refuses to abuse her body by feeding it too much food.

THIN -couragement _____

> Think of charting your hunger on a scale of 0–10. Zero is empty as when you're hungry and have physical hunger pangs. Five is comfortable, when you aren't either hungry or full. Seven is full—a slightly uncomfortable feeling—and ten is stuffed. To avoid overeating, eat only when your hunger number is 0 (hungry) and stop when it's at 5 (comfortable), before you are full.

Increase Muscle Mass

Your metabolism increases with an increase in muscle mass, so it's time to start an enthusiastic and lavish program for strength training. No matter what your age, you can produce quick and satisfying results when you pick up those weights and pump iron. Or you can also pump with a flex resistance band, stretch tubing, exercise machines, a body bar, or other interesting versions of free hand weights.

You can pump iron at a fitness center or a health club. Use the machines, use the free weights, or participate in some version of a "power-pump" fitness class. If you prefer a more serene environment, do your strength training with a Pilates class or a home video. You'll soon look as if you've lost weight, your clothes will fit better, and you'll lose weight faster.

Enjoy Your ZZZs

You need an adequate amount of sleep every night—about seven to eight hours—for your metabolism to run at optimal speed. Don't even think of cutting short your sleep time. No one is going to give you a badge of honor for sleeping fewer hours than your body requires. But you may inhibit your ability to lose weight if you don't sleep enough.

When you don't get enough sleep on a regular basis, your body's stress hormones, adrenaline and cortisol, increase. With an increase in stress hormones comes an increase in insulin levels. That means your body starts storing fat, which in turn slows down your metabolism. Avoid this vicious cycle.

Recent research has shown that sleep deprivation and jet lag disrupt a person's normal blood sugar levels and lead to cravings for white and fluffy starches—the high-glycemic kind you want to eat sparingly, if at all.

If sleep doesn't come easy to you, learn the basics of getting a good night's sleep. Sleep in a cool, dark, and quiet room. Avoid drinking caffeinated beverages before bedtime.

Go to bed at the same time every night. If you need more assistance or information, speak with your health practitioner.

> **Body of Knowledge** _____
>
> An easy way to determine how much sleep you need is to go to bed earlier and avoid setting your alarm clock. Instead, wake up naturally and note how long you slept. You need to do this every day for about a week to get a clear answer. For practical reasons, you might need to try this experiment during a vacation. After you've learned your natural sleep amount, schedule your life so that you get the ZZZs you need.

Balance Your Eating

Your body responds best when you eat balanced meals that contain protein, fat, and carbohydrates. When you're eating the low-glycemic way, carbs are an important and essential part of your meals. Don't exclude them; you could stall your metabolism. If you eat out-of-balance meals once in a while, don't worry; you can make up for it at the next meal. But if you avoid all carbs, all fats, or all protein repeatedly for a week or two, your body won't receive the nutrition it needs.

In addition, it's important to spread out the food you eat somewhat evenly throughout your day. Research shows that skipping meals increases your chance of becoming overweight. Eat breakfast, lunch, dinner, and a snack or two. Research also shows that people who eat breakfast are more likely to be their normal weight, and those who don't regularly eat breakfast are more likely to be overweight.

When you deprive yourself of proper nutrition, your body starts behaving as if it's in a famine situation and slows its metabolism; plus it starts storing fat. From the body's perspective, the advantage of slowing metabolism during a famine is to ensure that you have enough fuel on which to live. Fat has more energy per pound than muscle, so fat becomes an ideal fuel source.

Avoid High-Glycemic Foods

Those white, fluffy, or sticky high-glycemic foods slow you down and bring on late afternoon fatigue and midriff bloat. As you proceed with low-glycemic weight loss, you'll learn exactly what glycemic load your body can handle without gaining weight.

Perhaps you'll eat high-glycemic foods once in a while, but most likely, cookies and candy won't be a large part of your maintenance plan. It's impossible to tell you how much high-glycemic food your body can handle, because everyone's needs are different. But one thing is certain: your metabolism will be higher if you avoid them.

Drink Caffeine Cautiously

How caffeine affects your weight loss can vary. Some people can continue to drink a couple of cups of coffee or a caffeinated beverage every day and have great success on a low-glycemic weight-loss program. Others may find that it slows down progress.

Caffeine all by itself, even without cream and sugar, stimulates the production of insulin because it indirectly raises blood glucose levels. And, as stated previously, this increases fat storage and thwarts fat burning.

The only way to determine how caffeine works for you is to stop drinking it for a week or so and notice whether your weight loss increases. If you hit a weight-loss plateau, try eliminating caffeine. That might be enough to move you off the plateau.

Caffeine is in coffee and black and green teas, as well as in many soft drinks, both naturally and artificially sweetened.

Fewer Sweet Sips

Sipping on sweet-tasting beverages frequently can prevent or slow down weight loss. These include both naturally and artificially sweetened drinks. Additionally, avoiding artificially sweetened drinks such as "diet" sodas will help break the habit of longing for a sweet taste in your mouth.

One theory suggests that when your body tastes something sweet, it makes the assumption that food is on the way. For some biological reason not yet fully understood, your body thinks it's time to store fat. So enjoy your sweet-tasting beverages with a meal or all by themselves, but avoid sipping on them frequently all day long. Instead, sip on water. It's an all-time winner.

Calcium Intake

In studies, calcium has been shown to assist with weight loss, so make sure you eat plenty of foods that contain this bone-building nutrient. Calcium is found in salmon, sardines, seafood, broccoli, asparagus, almonds, cabbage, and dark-green, leafy vegetables.

Dairy products that contain calcium include milk, yogurt, and cheese. Some experts believe that the calcium in dairy products has limited bioavailability to the body; others think of dairy as a good source of bioavailable calcium. A study from Harvard shows that women who drink two or more glasses of milk a day have a higher risk of osteoporosis. For those reasons, be sure to eat plenty of other foods that contain calcium and don't rely solely on dairy products to supply all of your body's calcium needs.

Taking a calcium supplement may also be helpful. The adult body needs between 1,000 and 1,500 mg of calcium a day. Look for a supplement that offers bioavailable calcium.

Alcoholic Beverages

For the purposes of your glycemic index weight-loss program, alcohol is a food, contains calories, and needs to be noted in your daily food journal. A 3.5 ounce glass of white wine has 70 calories and one gram of carbohydrates. Just one ounce of 90-proof liquor has 73 calories and no carbs. And 12 ounces of beer has 146 calories and 13 grams of carbs.

The glycemic index of alcoholic beverages hasn't been tested with any accuracy because the glycemic index changes based on when the alcohol is consumed—before, during, or after a meal. We do know that alcohol can increase and then lower blood sugar levels, making them hard to predict. However, with all alcoholic beverages, even low-glycemic alcoholic beverages, you need to be careful. The body uses alcohol as fuel first, and only after the alcohol is used up does it obtain energy from your fat stores. This means that enjoying a glass or two of wine with dinner will stall your fat-burning process.

Another consideration is that alcohol is an appetite stimulant. Research shows that its effects vary with different people. Some people never notice an increase in appetite. Others notice an increased appetite effect for up to one week after that single glass of wine, which is exactly what you don't want.

And finally, alcoholic beverages stimulate production of the stress hormone cortisol. How much varies by frequency, amount, and of course, by person. High levels of cortisol are known to help pack on weight around your middle. They don't call 'em beer bellies for nothing.

The way to determine how alcohol affects your body is to keep a record of all the foods you eat and drink, including alcoholic beverages. Review your records for the week after you drank an alcoholic beverage. If you ate more food than normal for the next several days, alcohol could be an appetite stimulant for you. If a glass of wine stalls your progress or stimulates your appetite too much, pass on the alcohol in the future. It may be easiest to simply avoid alcoholic beverages altogether during your weight-loss program.

Wrong Weigh

You can now purchase low-carb beer, but should you? Probably not. Low-carb beer still contains alcohol, which elevates cortisol levels and insulin levels, while stimulating appetite. You'll drink fewer carbs than with regular beer, but you'll still need to contend with the fattening and appetite-stimulating qualities in beer.

Eat

If you're hungry and your hunger number is 0, and it's time for a meal or snack, go ahead and, by all means, eat. Don't skip meals thinking that it will help you lose weight. Skipping meals when you're hungry actually slows down your metabolism, because your body starts to use muscle tissue instead of fat for energy. So keep on eating regularly to keep your metabolism stoked.

THIN-couragement

One fabulous advantage of low-glycemic weight loss is that you're supposed to eat meals and snacks. You don't skip meals. You don't need to mess with liquid meals. And unlike diets that simply restrict calories without regard to food type, following a low-glycemic plan allows you to eat plenty of delicious foods and continue to lose weight.

Weight-Loss Blockers

Before you embark on your low-glycemic weight-loss program, you need to know that some medical conditions could prevent or stall your progress. If any of these apply to you, be sure to check with your doctor for advice.

Medications

Some prescription and over-the-counter medications can prevent or stall weight loss. They increase a person's metabolic resistance. These include the following:

◆ Steroids such as prednisone and, to a lesser degree, asthma inhalers

◆ Some anticonvulsants

◆ Some antidepressants

◆ Some hormone-replacement therapy medications

◆ Some birth control pills

◆ Insulin and insulin-stimulating medications

Not all drugs in these categories work the same way. If you suspect that your medication is thwarting your weight-loss efforts, talk with your doctor or pharmacist about other options. Discuss alternative choices, such as using nutritional supplements or lifestyle changes, to help you eliminate the need for these medications.

As you experience success with your glycemic index weight-loss program, your need for some medications, such as those for high blood pressure, may decrease or be eliminated.

Diet Sodas and Artificial Sweeteners

Yes, our dreams of a totally safe and healthy way to enjoy a sweet taste without calories have been crushed. Research shows that the artificial sweetener, Equal, also known as aspartame, stimulates sugar cravings and stimulates appetite. In addition, studies have shown that diet sodas increase the risk of metabolic syndrome and that people who regularly drink diet sodas weigh more than those who don't.

The safety of aspartame as a food product is also in doubt, and numerous complaints have been filed with the FDA about health complications due to drinking diet sodas.

The easiest way to deal with the controversy surrounding aspartame and diet soda is to avoid it. If you drink diet sodas regularly, find ways to reduce your consumption. Instead, drink purified water, water with lemon or lime, or mild herbal teas. This may not be easy at first, but the results are worth it—you'll find it easier to lose weight and to keep it off.

Many products other than diet sodas contain aspartame, like artificially sweetened yogurt, cereal, juice-type beverages, candy, and electrolyte beverages. Read labels carefully to make the best choices for your health.

The jury is out on the safety of the other popular artificial sweetener, sucralose. But stay posted, it's too soon to tell.

Yeast Infections

Chronic Candida albicans, or yeast infections, can prevent weight loss. Everyone's body contains both beneficial bacteria and yeast. It's only when the balance between the two is disrupted that a person's yeast overgrows to the point of a yeast infection. Yeast infections include such symptoms as rashes that itch, vaginitis, ringworm, athlete's foot, thrush, nail infections, and jock itch.

Yeast overgrowth increases appetite, especially for sweets and high-glycemic carbs. Those intense food cravings make it hard to follow a weight-loss program.

Often yeast infections are caused by the overuse of antibiotics, which have destroyed all the body's beneficial bacteria. Eliminating a yeast infection will help you lose weight. Many natural solutions can work but they may take several months to a year to totally clear your body of yeast overgrowth. Try these suggestions:

- Take an acidophilus nutritional supplement that contains bifidobacterium and bulgaricus. If you are sensitive to dairy, use a supplement that doesn't contain milk cultures. Take as directed.

- Mix up a powdered "greens" drink in water twice a day and drink. The drink can help produce an *alkaline-ash effect* and is filled with an abundance of beneficial phytonutrients, minerals, and vitamins. Yeast flourishes in an acidic environment, so by making the body slightly alkaline, the yeast dies off. Nutritionists frequently advocate that having a slightly alkaline body is healthier. You'll find "greens" drink mixes at the health-food store.

- Take cream of tartar several times a day. Stir 1–2 tsp. in a small amount of water. Chuck it and then follow with a glass of water. The cream of tartar is great at killing yeast, and you'll see why when you taste it. It's strong and very sour. But it works fabulously.

> **Glyco Lingo**
>
> An **alkaline–ash effect** occurs when the urine turns more alkaline. When the body is slightly alkaline, it's easier to maintain the proper bacteria-yeast balance level so that a person can reduce or eliminate urinary tract infections as well as yeast infections. You can test your urine pH with litmus strips available at pharmacies.

Clearing the body of yeast can be tricky and requires long-term determination. We suggest you do all of the above and stick with it. As you do, you'll lose weight and have more energy as your body comes into balance.

You can find other solutions for yeast infections at health-food stores. And if these suggestions don't work for you, you can also contact your health-care provider.

Low Thyroid

Your thyroid gland regulates your metabolism. If it's not functioning correctly, you could have metabolic resistance and be unable to lose weight. Other symptoms of an under-functioning thyroid include lethargy and fatigue, depression, sensitivity to cold, dry skin, chronic constipation, hair loss, poor memory, or elevated cholesterol levels.

If you suspect you have an underfunctioning thyroid, ask your doctor for a thyroid test to evaluate your T3, T4, and TSH levels. If they're low, you may need a prescription for a thyroid hormone, which is available as a naturally compounded medication called Armor or one that's not naturally compounded such as Synthroid, whichever you and your doctor prefer.

The Least You Need to Know

- Metabolic resistance is corrected through low-glycemic eating and lifestyle changes.

- Use strength training and aerobic exercise as ways to boost your basal metabolic rate.

- Increase your overall daily activity level so that you boost your metabolism and lift your mood.

- Make sure you get a good night's sleep to keep your metabolism high.

- A low thyroid hormone, yeast overgrowth, and some medications can stall or prevent weight loss.

The ABCs of Food and Eating

In This Chapter

- ◆ Using the Plate Method

- ◆ Choosing from the A-list

- ◆ Avoiding foods that flunk

- ◆ Eating for extra credit

As you read this book, you've noticed that food and eating "ain't what they used to be." Today, our knowledge about food and how it works in the body is far more advanced than even five years ago when we wrote the original version of this book.

The Plate Method of serving a meal is an excellent and easy way to know what to eat. Serve yourself and your family the portions we show you for proteins, carbohydrates, and fats, and you'll eat a nutritionally balanced meal.

As a further refinement, we show you how to factor the glycemic index along with the healthiest foods so you lose weight faster and keep it off easily. We'll use the grading system you're familiar with from your school days: A, B, C, and F along with extra credit. The more A's you choose and the more extra credit you eat, the easier and faster your weight loss.

You may be wondering if your appetite can be satisfied by eating A-sector foods. Because lower-glycemic foods generally stay in your stomach longer, are more bulky, and help keep blood sugar levels more stable, eating this way makes you more satisfied. We think you'll be pleasantly surprised. And your clothes will fit better.

THIN **-couragement**

> Take the Glycemic Index Food Source Chart with you to the grocery store. Purchase foods in the A sector, and you'll have the foods you need to be most successful with glycemic index weight loss.

Sizing Up Your Plate

The best way we've found to manage eating for glycemic index weight loss is by using the Plate Method. This is especially helpful if you're a visual person and have been known to eat based on what your eyes can take in rather than on what your stomach can accommodate.

The Plate Method is based on eating balanced meals for glycemic index weight loss. Here's what to put on your plate:

◆ Fill about half of your plate with nonstarchy vegetables such as green beans, peas, carrots, lettuce, cucumbers, tomatoes, zucchini, and onions. Except for beets, all nonstarchy vegetables are low glycemic. These types of veggies are lower in carbohydrate and calories than starchy vegetables.

◆ Fill about one quarter of your plate with low-glycemic starches, fruit, or dairy products. These three food groups are higher in carbohydrate and a little higher in calories than the nonstarchy veggies.

◆ One fourth of your plate is for lean protein, including meats, seafood, or poultry. That's enough room for about 3 to 4 ounces, or 15 to 20 grams.

◆ The remaining wedge of your plate, or about one eighth, is for healthy fats, such as olive oil, avocados, and nuts and seeds.

In actuality, your plate won't look exactly like this. Usually, the fats will be part of your foods, as dressing for your vegetables, or as nuts and seeds sprinkled over your salad. And, as you know, oils run and spread all over the other foods.

Use the Plate Method for teaching your children how to eat. Most likely, they'll relate well to the Plate Method. You can even ask them for food and meal suggestions to place on the plate.

The Plate Method really does work. Try it a few times so you can figure it out. All bets are off, though, if you go back for seconds. Serve food onto your plate with a sense of how it should look according to this formula. In no time at all you will be using it—even at challenging eating situations, such as at a buffet, a potluck dinner, or at Grandma's house.

> **Body of Knowledge**
>
> By filling almost half your plate with vegetables and having another quarter for fruit, you'll be sure to eat the recommended amount of 5 to 10 servings of vegetables and fruit every day.

Compare the size of a modern dinner plate to one in Grandma's china cupboard. A modern dinner plate has 36 square inches of surface area and an 11-inch diameter, compared to 33 on Grandma's with a 10-inch diameter. Simply by using a smaller plate, you'll eat less food at every meal. Eating all the food on those extra three square inches three times a day adds at least three more inches to your waistline over a year or two.

You may be wondering where dessert fits on the plate. Figure it goes into the spot reserved for fruit/starchy vegetables, or for fat. This reminds you to save room in your stomach for dessert, if you plan to eat some. It also helps keep your dessert portion size small but adequate.

Glycemic Index Food Source Chart

You know how important the glycemic index is to your weight loss and health. Now we want to add in another very significant component that will make a difference to your ultimate success: the natural and wholesome quality of the foods you eat.

From Farm or Factory to Your Plate

Some food arrives at the grocery store straight from the farm; some of it comes directly from a factory. Foods from both sources can be viable for your weight loss, so let's look at the differences so you can make the best choices.

Foods that come from the farm, such as vegetables, fruit, dairy, meat, fish, pure honey, nuts, seeds, herbs, and spices …

- Are natural and mostly low glycemic. Just a couple of vegetables and fruits are medium glycemic. Some starches, such as potatoes and rice, are high glycemic.

- Are nutrient-dense, meaning that they contain the highest concentration of vitamins, minerals, and antioxidants so you get the greatest value for your shopping dollar.

- Don't list manmade chemical ingredients on the nutritional label.

- Are biologically better because your body doesn't need to defend itself from the ingredients in these foods, with the possible exceptions of your allergies.

Foods that come from factories or food processing manufacturers may or may not be as wholesome as farm-sourced foods, but they can still be low glycemic. Foods at the right side of the Glycemic Index Food Source Chart go through more manufacturing steps and have more mystery ingredients than foods toward the left. At the far left are foods that are grown on farms, such as apples, beef, and lettuce. Easy ways to identify these foods are …

- The ingredient label lists artificial ingredients, such as preservatives, colorings, flavorings, MSG, dough tenderizers that aren't biologically friendly to your body and that may or may not ultimately be proved harmful.

- They may contain unpronounceable ingredients that may or may not be healthy for you.

- They may contain ingredients such as aspartame, an artificial sweetener, and others that actually cause a person to gain weight and increase the likelihood of having metabolic syndrome, the precursor to diabetes.

- They may contain trans fats or partially hydrogenated vegetable oil, which is known to cause heart disease.

- They may contain high-fructose corn syrup, which causes weight gain and obesity. Some cities are considering banning it.

- They may contain modified food starch or maltodextrins. These very high-glycemic fillers are found in low-fat processed foods and baked goods.

Virtually all of the above ingredients are considered to be toxins that your body needs to defend itself against. One way it does this is to store the toxins away from vital organs by placing them in body fat. If your body fat—think of it as a toxic waste dump for this explanation—gets too full of toxins, your body actually manufactures more fat in which to store the excess. Yes, this is scary. But it's avoidable and correctable.

Your best choice for your glycemic index weight-loss program is to purchase and eat farm-sourced foods and avoid factory-processed foods when you can.

THIN **-couragement** _____

> You can't avoid eating all factory-processed foods unless you never socialized, ate at restaurants, traveled on airplanes, or went to a sporting event. The real world and your real life necessitate eating factory-processed foods. That's okay. But as much as you can, eat farm-sourced foods.

The Best Food Choices

As you can see in the Glycemic Index Food Source Chart, it shows to how to make the best food selections.

Here are the main features:

◆ On the vertical axis is the glycemic index, ranging from low glycemic (0 to 55), to medium glycemic (56 to 69), on up to high glycemic (70 to 115).

◆ On the horizontal axis is a range of food categories: farm sourced; processed with nutritional value; processed with low or no nutritional value; and factory sourced with additives/mystery ingredients. The foods to the left are the most wholesome and natural, the foods to the right are the most highly processed and contain the most artificial ingredients.

◆ Each area of the graph contains a letter: A, B, C, A2, B2, C2, D, or F1, F2, and F3.

A-sector foods are the best for you to eat. They include low-glycemic farm-sourced foods, such as vegetables, fruits, meat, eggs, fish, poultry, most honey, legumes, sweet potatoes, thick-cut oatmeal, nuts, and seeds. Also included are minimally processed foods such as herbs, spices, pickles, horseradish, sun-dried tomatoes, most dried fruit, and other condiments. Dairy products such as milk, cheese, natural yogurt, and sour cream that don't contain additives and preservatives. Coffee and tea are also A foods.

B-sector foods are healthy for you, too, but medium glycemic. They include beets, fresh corn, basmati rice, cantaloupe, pineapple, wild rice, and stone-ground bread.

		Farm-Sourced Foods	Processed with Nutritional Value	Processed with Low-Nutritional Value	Factory-Source Foods-additives, "mystery" ingredients
High Glycemic		White potatoes Millet Popcorn Tapioca	Grape nuts Whole-wheat blended bread, finely milled	White bread Pretzels Rice cakes Bagel	Some protein bars Frozen desserts Gatorade Sodas Donuts Most boxed breakfast cereal French fries Crackers High-fructose corn syrup
		C	C2	D	F3
	70				
Medium Glycemic	69	Corn meal Raisins Figs Pineapple Wild rice	Some 100% grain breakfast cereals	Table sugar Instant oatmeal Brown sugar	Some candy Juice cocktail Some protein bars Potato chips
		B	B2	D	F2
	56				
Low Glycemic	55		Coarsely ground whole wheat bread Milk chocolate Ice cream Dark chocolate 100% Juice	Soy protein isolate	Soy milk Nonfat sugar-free fruit yogurts Trans fats Artificial sweeteners Diet Sodas
		A	A2	D	F1
	0				
		Farm-Sourced Foods	**Processed with Nutritional Value**	**Processed with Low-Nutritional Value**	**Factory-Source Foods-additives, "mystery" ingredients**

Glycemic Index Food Source Chart.

C-sector foods are high glycemic, but still farm sourced. They aren't great for low-glycemic eating, except in small amounts with foods that are low glycemic, They include white potatoes, millet, all-natural popcorn, parsnips, and rutabagas. Isn't it interesting that not many farm-sourced foods are high glycemic?

A2-sector foods are processed foods that contain great nutritional value and are low glycemic. They include 100-percent juice, coarsely ground whole-wheat and stone-ground breads, dark and milk chocolate, and pure, all natural ice cream.

B2-sector foods are natural, processed, medium-glycemic food. In this category are some 100-percent grain breakfast cereals.

C2-sector foods are natural, processed, and high glycemic. These include grape nuts and fluffy whole wheat bread made with finely-milled grain.

D-sector foods are processed foods with low to no nutritional value. They definitely aren't nutrient-dense, so you may not want to waste room in your stomach on D-sector foods when you could eat more nourishing fare. They aren't helpful for weight loss and health because they don't deliver value. They're far removed from being farm sourced.

Foods in the F-sector flunk. They're diet and health destroyers and need to be eaten with caution, if at all; preferably, you'd avoid them.

F1 foods flunk. Yes, they're low glycemic, but that's all they have going for them. Avoid these. They're full of mystery ingredients or artificial sweeteners. They include diet sodas, zero-calorie drink mixes, artificially sweetened diet foods, such as yogurt and cookies, soy milk, most beef jerky (unless it's totally natural), and corn dogs.

F2 foods also flunk. They're medium glycemic and full of mystery ingredients. These include frozen dinners, some candy, some protein bars, potato chips, juice cocktails, donuts, and corn chips.

F3 foods really flunk. They give you a double whammy of bad: high-glycemic foods filled with mystery ingredients. No amount of extra credit can make up for eating too many F3 foods. These include frozen soy desserts, sugary boxed cereals, sodas, colas, electrolyte-replenishment drinks like Gatorade, high-caffeine sodas, popsicles,

Wrong Weigh

The Glycemic Index Food Source Chart is a guideline for you—don't let it make you rigid in your food choices. Yes, eat A-grade foods most of the time, but don't pass up a piece of wedding cake or a slice of pizza in an effort to be perfect. Perfection doesn't work in weight loss or in life; flexibility and "going with the flow" do.

candy (such as jelly beans), many protein bars and power bars, French fries, and many other "treat" foods.

Using the Chart

The chart simplifies food shopping, menu planning, and eating. Eat mostly A-grade foods. Plan your meals around them. Seek them out at restaurants. Yes, even fast-food restaurants offer some A-grade foods. You can always order a burger, hold the bread, and add a salad.

Eat B-grade foods occasionally, and some C-grade foods. If you love potatoes, balance the potatoes with low-glycemic foods and sour foods at that meal, and you'll probably be fine. "Probably" means based on your current level of health, your personal biology, and your weight-loss goals.

Take the chart with you to the grocery store, and you'll notice that you'll be doing most of your shopping around the perimeter—in the produce, meats, seafood, and dairy sections. You'll be stepping into the aisles mostly for baking supplies, spices and condiments, coffee, tea, and household staples.

THIN-**couragement**

Most fine restaurants pride themselves in offering fresh and natural ingredients so you can enjoy their varied and creative meals with confidence. And if in doubt, ask the chef. He or she may be delighted to discuss ingredients and food preparation with you.

Extra Nutritional Credit

Some foods and ways of eating are like the frosting on the cake. You'll be topping off your eating choices with an enlightened approach to your weight loss. Follow these extra-credit guidelines to reach your goals:

1. Take 1 to 2 tablespoons of fish oil or cod liver oil every day. Check with your doctor if you're on blood-thinning medications.

2. Eat sour or acidic-tasting foods with each meal.

3. Eat 9 to 10 servings of vegetables or fruit daily. That's three per meal.

4. Drink up to eight glasses of purified water a day.

5. Eat cold-water fish two to three times every week.

6. Eat hot chili peppers and spicy food often. The hot spices aid in weight loss.

7. Take a calcium supplement daily.

8. Take vitamin D₃ every day, either from cod liver oil or as a nutritional supplement, or spend 15 minutes in the sun every day with your skin exposed (arms and legs are enough).

Isn't it amazing that losing weight is about eating delicious and interesting food with mindfulness and love? It's no longer about deprivation and isolation.

The Least You Need to Know

- Use the Plate Method for filling your plate at mealtimes and for teaching your children how to eat.

- By using the Plate Method, you'll be limiting your portions without weighing and measuring.

- Farm-sourced foods are more beneficial for weight loss than factory-sourced foods.

- The Glycemic Index Food Source Chart shows you how to make healthy and wholesome food choices that work for glycemic index weight loss.

- Add a final touch of wise and enlightened eating to your daily food intake by following the 8-step Extra Nutritional Credit recommendations.

Chapter 8

Beginning Your Glycemic Index Weight-Loss Program

In This Chapter

- Choosing your best time
- Determining your goal size and weight
- Charting your progress
- Using a weight-loss journal

Now that you know the basics of glycemic index weight loss, you're probably excited about getting started. However, you might have some reservations about starting yet another diet program. By now, you may have been on enough diets to know that losing weight isn't exactly a cakewalk. You'll be making lifestyle changes, but you'll also be learning all about your body's biology in relation to carbohydrates and weight loss. This information will serve you well the rest of your life as you become one of those people who are naturally thin with a healthy and fit physique.

Can you do this? Of course you can! Thousands of people have been successful at not only losing weight, but also keeping it off. As you know, the real success isn't losing the weight; it's staying at your ideal size for life.

Right this moment, tell yourself that you will be "healthy, happy, and the size I want to be." Then read on for some tips and tools to help you make that statement come true!

Timing Is Everything

In one sense, any time is the best time to lose weight. You don't want to wait one more second to make your excess weight disappear. Impatience can be an important advantage in weight loss. It means you're ready to do what it takes.

On the other hand, some times in life are better than others. You can set yourself up for success by reading through the following statements. If one or more are true for you, now may *not* be your best time to jump into a glycemic index weight-loss program:

♦ You need to lose weight quickly to look great at an upcoming event, such as a wedding or high school reunion. This kind of motivation often backfires, leading to yo-yo dieting, which never works. Think of glycemic index eating as a way of life, not as a means to quick weight loss. However, an important upcoming event could be the positive trigger that gets you started successfully on a long-term glycemic index weight-loss program.

♦ You don't have time in your life right now to give glycemic index weight loss the time and attention it requires and you deserve.

♦ Your friend, spouse, doctor, or parent is urging you to lose weight. We applaud their suggestions to you, but unless you really want to lose weight, you aren't likely to succeed.

THIN -couragement

You can eat based on the glycemic index if you are pregnant or nursing, but you'll need a higher glycemic load. Although eating mostly low glycemic will benefit you and your baby, it is not recommended to start a weight-loss program during pregnancy or the first four months of nursing.

On the other hand, you're in great shape to get started if …

♦ You're starting a glycemic index weight-loss program of your own free will.

♦ You're committed to doing whatever it takes because you really want to live at your ideal size.

♦ You have the dedication and freedom to eat mostly low-glycemic foods.

♦ You want to go the distance, knowing that on any weight-loss program it can take months to lose weight and the rest of your life to keep it off.

Good for you! You are in an ideal situation and state of mind to be successful, so let's get started.

Measurement Selection

You have many choices for measuring your progress. Although most people use weight scales to measure their progress, some are so turned off by the anxiety of stepping on the scales after many years of dieting that they prefer a different approach. We don't favor scales. Here is a variety of other measurement choices:

♦ **Monitor your measurements.** Before you start on your program, use a tape measure and record your chest or bust, waist, hip, upper thigh, and upper arm measurements. Then once a week or once every other week, take your measurements until you get to your ideal size. Then update them every month thereafter. If you want, set personal goals that outline what you want your ideal size and measurements to be.

♦ **Choose your ideal size.** If you're a man who felt great when you wore a size 36-inch belt, set that as your goal. If you're a woman who yearns to be a size 8 again, set that as your goal. Find a pair of jeans that you would love to fit into. Try them on every week as you progress through the program. You'll know you've reached your goal right away when you can zip them up comfortably and also when you can sit down in them. Keep those jeans for life. Try them on every month or two to make sure you're staying at your ideal size.

♦ **Determine your ideal body fat percentage.** Lowering your body fat percentage is a healthful choice, so measuring it regularly is a good guide to overall health and fitness. You can have your body fat measured at a fitness center, health club, or health fair. There are many ways to measure body fat, such as with calipers, with a bioimpedance machine, and with underwater body measuring. All can meet your purpose, which is to measure the decrease in your body fat as you lose weight and tone up. The important thing is to have your body fat measured the same way every time. You'll get a more reliable measure of improvement.

Measure your body fat percentage at the start of your program and every two to three months thereafter.

Here's a chart that shows body fat percentages. Set your goal body fat percentage based on these ranges:

Status	Women	Men
Athlete level	17	10
Lean	17–22	10–15
Normal	22–25	15–18
Above Normal	25–29	18–20
Overweight	29–35	20–25
Obese	over 35	over 25

The lower percentages are usually found in highly athletic individuals. If your body fat percentage is within the ideal range for your age, you don't need to be too concerned about your actual weight, because you'll look great and possess a higher metabolic rate. In other words, you could weigh more than you want, but look and feel great.

◆ **Use the scale.** Weigh yourself once a week—no more—and preferably on the same day at the same time each week. Stepping on the scales daily isn't a good indicator of your progress because your weight can fluctuate too much from one day to the next and for seemingly no reason. Keep a notepad near the scales and record each week's weight. If you follow an exercise program, and we strongly advise you to get plenty of exercise, you'll be increasing your muscle mass. Muscle weighs more than fat, so your weight could be higher than you were expecting, but you'll be fitting comfortably into your clothes. This is actually a good situation because it means your basal metabolic rate is also higher. And the higher your metabolic rate, the easier it is for you to lose weight.

◆ **Calculate your body mass index (BMI).** This number is used by government agencies and health-care practitioners to determine whether a person is over-weight or obese. If your BMI is between 25 and 29, you're considered to be overweight. If it's over 30, you're considered to be obese. You can use the chart that follows to determine your BMI.

BMI (kg/m2)	19	20	21	22	23	24	25	26	27	28	29	30	35	40
Height (in.)					*Weight (lb.)*									
58	91	96	100	105	110	115	119	124	129	134	138	143	167	191
59	94	99	104	109	114	119	124	128	133	138	143	148	173	198
60	97	102	107	112	118	123	128	133	138	143	148	153	179	204
61	100	106	111	116	122	127	132	137	143	148	153	158	185	211
62	104	109	115	120	126	131	136	142	147	153	158	164	191	218
63	107	113	118	124	130	135	141	146	152	158	163	169	197	225
64	110	116	122	128	134	140	145	151	157	163	169	174	204	232
65	114	120	126	132	138	144	150	156	162	168	174	180	210	240
66	118	124	130	136	142	148	155	161	167	173	179	186	216	247
67	121	127	134	140	146	153	159	166	172	178	185	191	223	255
68	125	131	138	144	151	158	164	171	177	184	190	197	230	262
69	128	135	142	149	155	162	169	176	182	189	196	203	236	270
70	132	139	146	153	160	167	174	181	188	195	202	207	243	278
71	136	143	150	157	165	172	179	186	193	200	208	215	250	286
72	140	147	154	162	169	177	184	191	199	206	213	221	258	294
73	144	151	159	166	174	182	189	197	204	212	219	227	265	302
74	148	155	163	171	179	186	194	202	210	218	225	233	272	311
75	152	160	168	176	184	192	200	208	216	224	232	240	279	319
76	156	164	172	180	189	197	205	213	221	230	238	246	287	328

The BMI is an excellent measurement, but it has some limitations. The formula penalizes someone who has lots of lean muscle, such as body builders and athletes. That's not good. If your body fat is low and your muscle mass is high, your BMI would put you into the overweight or obese category. In other words, highly muscled individuals who are definitely not overweight often have a high BMI because muscle weighs more. Most of us wish we had this problem! Any and all of these measurement gauges work. Which one you choose depends on what feels best to you. You can use all of them, one of them, or a combination. But by all means, measure your progress.

THIN -couragement

Scales only measure your specific gravity in relationship to the earth. They don't tell you how you look and feel. Most dieters who are hooked on "weighing in" every day don't take into account the fact that exercise will make you look better but may actually make you weigh more. That's because muscle weighs three times as much as fat for the same amount of volume. So don't rely on the scale as the only measuring stick of success. You want to reduce your size, so burning up bulky fat (which weighs less) and building lean muscle (which weighs more) is the way to do it. The scale can't give you a true indication of your progress.

Setting Your Goal

The best way to set your weight or size goal is to be both realistic and optimistic. Realistic so that you can reach your goal, and optimistic to stay motivated. You never know what you can really achieve until you try your best!

If you are a woman who is 5'10" with a large frame, setting your goal as "I want to wear a size 6" is probably unrealistic. But perhaps a size 10 or 12 (maybe even size 8) is within the range of possibility. On the other hand, it would be a mistake for this woman to talk herself out of a size 10 or 12 and instead shoot for a size 16 if she really wants to recapture her youthful college-age silhouette. Her optimism to become a size 10 or 12 could actually propel her to reach her goal. You can always change your goal as you near your ideal size. And believe it or not, you do have a choice as to what size you'll be.

Be realistic about how long it will take for you to lose weight. This is *so* important! You already know your excess weight won't melt off overnight. In truth, it likely won't all come off in three months. Instead, plan on losing one or two pounds a week, or a dress or belt size every two months. You may progress faster or slower, so use these as estimates only. If this seems discouraging, just know that weight loss takes as long as it takes, but the end result—your ideal size—is yours to keep.

What's your hurry? Predictably, 9 times out of 10, yo-yo dieters are in a hurry to lose pounds, even lots of pounds. As Shakespeare would say, "That way lies madness." You didn't gain those 20 pounds in two months; don't try to lose them in two months. Although some people do successfully lose weight quickly, it's not the norm. Nor is it better. Slow, steady weight loss is more likely to last for the long term. And you won't be as tempted to quit just because you don't see huge reductions right away.

Set Up Your Daily Journal

After you have determined how to measure your progress, you need somewhere to track it. Purchase a journal or a spiral-bound notebook to use as your journal for your glycemic index weight loss. Depending on the amount of weight you want to lose and the length of time it takes, you might fill up several volumes.

Begin your journal by writing out your start date, your current size and weight, and your goals. Mark a section for recording your body's progress, another section to serve as a food diary, and a third section to track your exercise sessions.

Consider your journal to be very personal. After all, it's your history and it's also going to be filled with information that records your progress.

> ## THIN-couragement
>
> A daily journal is really, really valuable. Don't avoid creating one just because it seems like a hassle. Researchers have shown that people who record their food intake lose more weight than those who don't. You will learn a lot from your journal. By the way, don't "cheat" in your journal; it's for your eyes only.

Your Daily Records

Record your food intake every day. That means everything you ate or drank except for water. Set up a page for each day and have it look like this:

Date: include the day of the week

Time: record time of day

Beginning Hunger Number: on a scale of 0–10, 0 being empty, 5 being comfortable, and 10 being stuffed, what's your hunger number before you start to eat? Ideally, your stomach hunger would be a 0, zero.

Food or Beverage: list the foods or beverages you consumed.

Amount: list the amount but please don't weigh and measure. Instead, you can record the amounts using more general terms such as a cup of soup, one slice of pizza topping without crust, large chef salad, etc.

GI Rating: use the categories high, medium, low, or very low to indicate the GI rating.

Optional: list the glycemic load of the item. This is optional based on whether you choose the Keep It Simple or the Comprehensive program as defined in Chapter 10.

Ending Hunger Number: when you've completed eating the meal, what's your stomach hunger number? Ideally, it's a 5—you're not feeling hungry, and you're also not feeling full. If it's above a 5, wait until your stomach is once again at 0 before you eat again.

You'll love the results of using a daily food journal to stay on track. The format invites self-discipline and forgiveness. Continue your journal until you attain your ideal size. After that, you may choose to use it from time to time if you sense that you're regaining some weight. If this happens, *do not* delay. Open up the journal the day you sense your jeans are getting tight. They'll be looser within a week.

The Least You Need to Know

♦ Set a time to begin your glycemic index weight loss that fits into your schedule and personal needs.

♦ Choose your goal size and weight carefully, using pounds, how your jeans fit, body fat percentages, or BMI.

♦ Use a daily food diary to record your food intake and to keep you on track.

Chapter 9

Get Your Mind Aligned

In This Chapter

- Harnessing your mental powers
- Utilizing the power of weight-loss affirmations
- Banishing past weight-loss failures
- Connecting with new eating behaviors
- Feeling thin

Attempting any weight-loss program can be either inspiring or depressing. The difference depends on you and your attitude. Based on all the scientific research, glycemic index weight loss is extraordinarily effective and safe. Yet even on a low-glycemic plan, some people succeed at losing weight and maintaining their ideal size for life, and some people don't.

You want to be one of those who succeed. You want to be someone who lives a healthy life at your ideal size. So it's important to use all the tools available, including the power of your mind.

In this chapter, you learn how to actively employ your innate mental power throughout your entire weight-loss and maintenance experience. It's readily available, it's totally free, and it will do exactly what you want it to do. All you need is to tell your mind what to think and your feelings what to feel.

Your Private Weight-Loss Ally

Many diet programs, this book included, tell you exactly what and when to eat to lose weight. Most teach you all you need to know about how your biology works to gain, store, and lose fat. But you need more. Your ultimate success depends on one factor of your biology seldom mentioned in any dieting or weight-loss program—your mind.

Your mind is your innate mental power. The power of your mind is far greater than your willpower and self-discipline. In fact, right now your willpower and self-discipline are likely strong enough for you to start on a low-glycemic weight-loss program.

You need to follow up your determination with positive thinking and a positive mental attitude. Positive thinking isn't simply a good idea for motivation, it's a necessity. Self-talk is actually a self-fulfilling prophecy. What you think you'll achieve is exactly what you will achieve. But first you need to take an honest look at your inner thoughts about your weight and your weight-loss history.

)HIN(-couragement

Time and again, we hear of athletes who first visualize their competitive goals, then talk positively about their goals, and ultimately reach their goals. The same can be true for you in your weight-loss efforts.

The Ghost of Weight-Loss Past

Whether you call them ghosts or skeletons, after years of dealing with weight issues, you are haunted by past failures. Unfortunately, they can seem to predict your future, and that prediction can be anything but positive, uplifting, and inspiring. In fact, it can be bleak. The first step in using your mental power to reach your goals is to identify your negative self-talk.

You might already doubt yourself with such questions and statements as …

◆ What makes me think I can succeed this time?

◆ How can I possibly deprive myself of all my favorite junk foods? Not just for now, but forever?

◆ I have fat genes.

◆ Everyone in my family is fat.

◆ I have no willpower.

◆ I might lose my friends if I lose weight.

◆ It's too expensive to eat low-glycemic foods.

◆ I've lost and gained the same 50 pounds over and over again.

◆ I hate vegetables.

◆ As I get older, I'm just naturally getting bigger.

◆ I was overweight as a child, so I don't know what it would be like not to be fat.

You get the dialogue. It goes on and on, and you can probably think of many more statements or questions to add to the previous list. In a sense, all negative self-talk has an element of truth to it. But negative self-talk is also deceptive, because these thoughts are the very thoughts that have held you and your body back from living at your ideal size. They've literally made themselves true.

Wrong Weigh _____

Avoid the very real temptation to feel guilty and blame yourself if you don't stick to your glycemic index weight-loss eating plans. Losing weight is at best an imperfect process. If you overeat or eat incorrectly, forgive yourself so that you banish guilt and discouragement. Instead, refocus your energy and eat according to plan at your next meal.

After identifying the negative self-talk about your size, weight, and eating, the next step is to convert those statements into what you want to be true.

Creating New Thoughts

For every negative statement of self-talk, there is an opposite, positive statement. Your mission is to turn around your thoughts so that you actually affirm what you want.

For example, the opposite positive of "I hate vegetables" is "I love vegetables." Now, now, instead of saying "Oh, yuck" to yourself, think again. If you continue to hate vegetables, this low-glycemic weight-loss program is going to be painful, unpleasant, and short-lived. If you essentially convince yourself that you love vegetables, however, you're going to love eating the low-glycemic way.

Although it might seem untrue, you can change virtually any thought you have, and only you can do it. The same goes for losing weight. No one else can do it for you.

ᘜHIᑎ **-couragement**

If you tell yourself that you love vegetables, your subconscious will eventually come to believe this. You're going to find yourself requesting a double order of broccoli or zucchini at restaurants. And, of all wonders, they'll be satisfying and delicious.

The same can be true for any thought. Take the statement "It's too expensive to eat low-glycemic foods." Turn it around to the opposite positive. "Eating low-glycemic foods fits well within my food budget." Only then will you discover that it can actually cost less to eat low-glycemic foods—such as a side salad at a fast-food drive-through rather than a pricier burger, fries, and soda.

The main benefit to rewriting the negative statements into positive ones is that you gain the power and momentum to reach your goals. And you'll eventually do it with more ease, less frustration, and more confidence.

In the beginning pages of your weight-loss journal, write down your biggest objections and self-doubts. Then underneath each one write the opposite positive. Review the list whenever you feel discouraged or want to toss out the cabbage or green beans and head to the neighborhood bakery for éclairs and crème puffs.

Your Personal Affirmations

As you begin to make the necessary mental shifts in self-talk, you need a concise set of personal affirmations. Affirmations are forward-thinking statements written in the present tense.

You can choose from the following or make up a set of your own:

◆ I enjoy living and eating based on the glycemic index.

◆ I am now at my ideal size and I easily stay at my ideal size for life. (Use this affirmation even if you aren't already at your ideal size. You are actually programming your subconscious to do the inner work to get you there.)

◆ I am now a naturally thin person and I wear a size _____. (Insert your ideal size.)

◆ I am now enjoying the health and energy benefits of eating the low-glycemic way.

◆ I am comfortable and safe at my ideal size.

◆ I am successful and happy at my ideal size.

◆ I love, honor, and appreciate my body.

- I enjoy lavish exercise.

- I exercise vigorously three to four times a week.

- I enjoy eating and preparing low-glycemic meals and snacks.

- I am in harmony with being at my ideal size.

- I easily eat low-glycemic meals when dining out, on vacations, and when traveling.

- My body feels great when I eat low-glycemic foods.

And try this one on for size: I have skinny genes. Or is it skinny jeans? Of course, it's both!

Affirmations are powerful tools. On a low-glycemic eating program, affirmations are as essential as meats and vegetables.

But affirmations are only powerful if you use them. After you have a complete list, you need to start working with them on a daily basis. Remember, it doesn't matter whether your list seems within the realm of possibility. In fact, it probably shouldn't be. Quite honestly, your affirmations should sound far-fetched and outrageous. If you were already living them, you would already be at your ideal size.

> **Body of Knowledge**
>
> You can use affirmations for other aspects of your life. Use them for success with your work, relationships, and health. Just be sure that your affirmations are positive, present tense, and that they preferably start with "I am."

The first time you read through your affirmations, focus on each one and feel the positive feelings of having it be true for you. Feel what it feels like to be naturally thin, to maintain your ideal size for life, and to enjoy exercise. Strongly link your positive emotional feelings to each affirmation. Then, each time you read through your affirmations or say them aloud, evoke the emotion once again. The mind-emotion link makes your affirmations work faster and stick better.

Keep your list with you. Write affirmations in your journal, post them on your computer, and key them into your PDA. Post them in the kitchen and on your desk at work. Record them on your computer, download the recording to your iPod or MP3 player, and listen to them throughout the day. And if your car often serves as an office away from home, post them on the dashboard.

At least once a day, and preferably twice, say each affirmation out loud. Set aside your incredulity and just say them. You'll soon get in the flow of their power, and eating the low-glycemic way will become second nature to you. Your results will prove your former inner-self doubts wrong.

A Treasure Map

Living at your ideal size has probably been a goal of yours for a long time. Attainment is within your grasp. Setting up visual cues supports your goal. Do this by creating a "treasure map." It can be as elaborate or as simple as you like.

Start with poster board or devote a wall to your treasure map. A simple treasure map might contain just one image—a picture that represents you at your ideal size. It might be a picture of you in earlier days when you were at your ideal size. It can also be a picture of a thin man or woman cut out from a magazine, perhaps with your face superimposed on the image.

THIN -couragement

As you put together your treasure map, remember that you're in this for the long run. Add pictures of what you'll be doing next year, and the year after that, and also add pictures of the low-glycemic foods that you enjoy the most.

Your treasure map can consist of one or more images in different locations, or you can create an elaborate, poster-sized treasure map with pictures of yourself, your favorite low-glycemic foods, and even pictures of a dream beach vacation you want to take.

Paste a motivating picture or pictures in your journal. You might also want to paste in a "before" photo and "progress" photos. Paste a motivational picture wherever you'll see it frequently. The bathroom mirror is a good location, and you can use the picture as a desktop image on your computer.

A treasure map keeps you focused on your goal and makes living through the details of getting there a whole lot easier.

Real-Time Concerns

Even though glycemic index weight loss is a terrific choice for weight loss, a time might come when you doubt yourself and your program. Don't let doubts and discouragements prevent you from attaining your ideal size. Instead, use them as a springboard.

First, recognize that the part of you that's speaking at the moment is the Ghost of Weight-Loss Past. This scary ghost comes from your mischievous brain remembering past emotions and frustrations—which is really what it's programmed to do. So it's okay to acknowledge what that old ghost has to say, but it's not okay to act on what it says. Don't let past failures dictate your present and future.

Instead, ignore that ghost for a moment and ask yourself—your current powerful, committed, and enthusiastic self—what you want. The answer is to attain your ideal size and to go the distance. Your powerful self can turn around the situation right then and there by saying aloud your list of affirmations.

This is exactly why you need to keep your affirmations close at hand all the time, because you never know when that ghost is going to appear.

Modeling "Thin" Behaviors

You didn't become overweight by eating like a thin person. No one does. Right now, social scientists who study weight issues and obesity are turning their attention to the 35 percent of the U.S. population who are naturally at their ideal size. To give others a model to go by, these researchers are looking for the behavior patterns of people who have been successful in controlling their weight.

Here's a list of "thin" behaviors to model:

- Eat when your stomach is truly hungry (at a zero) and avoid eating when prompted by television advertising, donut day at the office, or other feeding opportunities. After a few times of saying "no," it becomes remarkably easier.

- Sit down when you eat. Rather than stand at the kitchen counter or over the stove, pull up a seat and relax enough to savor your food.

- Rather than snack mindlessly when you're watching television or working on your computer, keep food in the kitchen and away from entertainment centers and your work space when at home.

- At the office, completely clear out high-glycemic snacks from your desk, and never eat in your car unless the car is stopped and you have no other alternatives. Pack along healthy snacks for your work breaks: peanut butter, dried fruit and nuts, packages of cheese, dark chocolate, olives, wholesomely prepared beef jerky, tuna in small bags.

- Develop an aversion to overeating and that stuffed feeling in your stomach.

- When you go out to eat, split an entrée with your spouse, children, or whomever you are with. No one needs that much food—the serving size is way bigger than your fist—it may be bigger than three or four fists. (One fist is a meal.) And, of course, you can split a dessert four or five ways. You'll find that a bite or two can be just as satisfying, and perhaps even more satisfying, than the whole piece of cheesecake or mud pie—both of which are usually medium glycemic.

◆ When dining alone, ask for a half-serving, or only eat half—or less—and take the remaining food home. (You can also ask for a take-home box at the start of the meal and immediately put half away. Out of sight, out of mind, and best of all, the food's not in your mouth.)

◆ Eat slowly. Don't rush. Savor your food.

◆ Avoid making eating your entertainment or your therapist. Instead, develop healthier outlets for fun and comfort.

◆ Become a picky eater and never make a point of cleaning your plate. Eat what you need to eat. Remember, cleaning your plate is fattening.

As you adopt these behaviors, you'll find that it's easier to go the distance with glycemic-index weight loss and you'll have fewer moments of missing "the good old overeating days."

The Top Ten List for Weight Loss

Our "Top Ten" list supports the inner you as you make outer changes. Losing weight is a significant undertaking. It changes the way you think, the way you interact with others, and even the structure of your lifestyle. Use this list to keep yourself centered and happy during the days, weeks, and years ahead.

1. Understand that food is not magic—it can only satisfy stomach hunger and sustain life. It has no power to make you happy, mend a broken heart, or make a loved one call.

2. Don't ever say, "Do I look fat?"

3. Don't talk about your weight-loss program unless you want to be boring or want to create resentment and jealously in others. And especially, don't talk about food choices, eating, or weight loss when eating with others.

4. Don't let "just this once" become a daily way of eating.

5. Find positive, inspiring, and uplifting projects to replace having a weight problem.

6. Don't replace the problem of overeating with another addictive-type problem such as spending, smoking, or drinking.

7. Don't be afraid of food or eating. It will make you fat. Likewise, don't be afraid of regaining your lost weight. You know how to keep it off. Fear can drive compulsive behavior and overeating.

8. Relax to eat, don't eat to relax.

9. Don't exercise more so you can eat more.

10. Never, never, never, never, never overeat.

If you have other pet peeves about yourself or others who are losing weight, add them to this list. You need all the support you can get, and you yourself are your biggest fan and strongest supporter.

Food and eating are powerful. We need them to survive, but overdoing them creates weight gain and chronic disease. Use this list to help you stay in balance and to walk lightly along the path to living at your ideal size.

The Least You Need to Know

◆ Your mental power is a terrific asset for losing weight and keeping it off.

◆ Use affirmations to harness the power of your mind and to stay on track with your low-glycemic weight-loss program.

◆ Attach strong positive emotions and feelings to each affirmation.

◆ Chart your weight-loss progress by using posters and graphs.

◆ Model the behaviors of thin people to jump-start your program.

Your Choice: Two Glycemic Index Weight-Loss Programs

In This Chapter

◆ Discovering the Keep It Simple program

◆ Learning the Comprehensive program

◆ Making adjustments

◆ Maintaining your weight loss

There's no time like the present. That is especially true when embarking on a new eating plan based on the glycemic index.

If you've read this far, you're ready to start. You understand the basics of the glycemic index. You've learned some fundamental aspects of weight loss. And you're determined to successfully lose weight and keep it off.

In this chapter, we give you two methods for using the glycemic index to lose weight. The first program is simple and easy because you don't need to count or calculate; however, your food choices are somewhat more limited. The second program is more detailed and specific, but it offers you more food choices. You can decide which one works best for you.

Both choices give you room to savor and enjoy delicious foods while you keep your fat-burning mechanism revved up, allowing you to lose weight safely and easily.

Don't be intimidated by the glycemic index, it's quite friendly. It works because it's patterned after how your body's biology works. As you eat based on the glycemic index, your eating patterns will be more aligned with your DNA and your biology. You'll be living and eating in harmony with yourself.

Two Glycemic Eating Programs

Forget what you've heard about *induction phases*, or three-phase weight-loss programs. With glycemic index weight loss, there is only one phase. This means that you'll use the same program to begin losing weight and to continue your weight loss. You may want to adjust the program as you move into lifelong weight maintenance and understand how different foods and glycemic loads affect your body.

> **Glyco Lingo**
>
> An **induction phase** is a standard part of some weight-loss programs. In the two-week induction phase, a person eats strictly limited amounts of carbohydrates, most of which are "free vegetables." Induction phase eating is not balanced, not necessary for weight loss, and happily not included in a glycemic index weight-loss program.

Eating based on the glycemic index can be intricate and complex or it can be very simple. If you don't have time in your life to count, weigh, and measure, use the first program—Keep It Simple. If you prefer a more rigorous program, use the second program—Comprehensive. Either way, you'll be able to reach your weight-loss goals.

Program One—Keep It Simple

The first program will work best for you if you have always wanted a weight-loss program that's stunningly simple. Here are some other ways to know if you want simple and easy:

◆ You don't have time to calculate glycemic load.

◆ You are very busy or live a high-stress life.

◆ You frequently eat at restaurants, travel, or lead a hectic social life.

◆ You are allergic to or have food sensitivities to wheat or gluten or you have *celiac disease*. Although these aren't common health conditions, if you need to avoid wheat or gluten and need to lose weight, the Keep It Simple program will work for you.

Glyco Lingo _____

Celiac disease is a chronic digestive disorder that's caused by intolerance to gluten. Gluten is found in wheat, spelt, rye, oats, and barley. Most common in Caucasians of European descent, people with celiac disease need to avoid eating foods that contain gluten, because it can be life-threatening.

◆ You cook for a full family—spouse, children, and others.

If "keeping it simple" is how you wish you could live, choose this program.

What to Eat

First of all, you'll need to be able to assess the glycemic index rating of a carbohydrate simply by looking at a food. Don't worry, we do this for ourselves all the time. Here are the important guidelines we use:

White or fluffy makes you puffy. Avoid eating white or fluffy foods most of the time. This includes most cakes, breads, bagels, crackers, rice crackers, popcorn, cookies, donuts, muffins, boxed breakfast cereals, non-cooked breakfast cereals, chocolate cake, pasta, pancakes, French toast, wheat bread, rice, cinnamon rolls, pretzels, white potatoes, quinoa, and puffed rice and wheat. Add in tortillas, corn chips, and potato chips.

We've included soy protein isolate as a white or fluffy food because it's a highly processed form of soy. It's best to eat soy as edamame or tofu.

Exceptions to this rule are real crunchy stone-ground bread, Irish cut oatmeal, pasta cooked until just barely al dente, basmati rice, and sourdough bread. The following foods when cooked, chilled, and eaten when cold or room temperature contain resistant starches: white potatoes, corn, barley, rice, yams, and bananas. The resistant starches make the foods lower glycemic than before they were cooked and chilled.

Other exceptions include the recipes at the back of this book and in our cookbook, *The Complete Idiot's Guide Glycemic Index Cookbook*. We've carefully designed desserts, breads, and grains to be low glycemic.

If it's sticky, be real picky. In other words, don't eat sticky foods unless they're really worth it and you have room in your stomach. Sticky foods include caramel apples, chocolate bonbons, lollypops, popsicles, caramel corn, mud pie, cheesecake, pudding, thick white sauces, chocolate and butterscotch sauce, ice cream sundaes and shakes, toffee, brownies, and pies.

Sticky foods may contain lots and lots of sugar or, if they're a factory-sourced food, worse: high-fructose corn syrup along with artificial colorings, flavorings, and preservatives. If you simply have to eat a sticky food, it's best to eat it with a meal, rather than apart from other food.

Some recipes at the back of this book and in our cookbook offer sweet sticky-type foods that are low glycemic, so if your sweet tooth needs satisfaction, cook up one of those.

Vegetables are your friend. Eat two to three servings of vegetables or fruit at every meal. That's six to nine servings daily.

Most vegetables and fruit are low glycemic, but don't worry if they aren't. You can enjoy all, provided that you don't overload on fruit. Limit fruit servings to a max of ½ your daily total servings. So if you're eating nine servings of vegetables and fruit daily, have four servings of fruit.

A serving of vegetables is ½ cup cooked or 1 cup raw. A small apple is one serving, a large apple is two servings.

Eat high-quality, complete protein at each meal or three times a day. Yes, you need complete nutrition at each meal, including breakfast. High-quality complete protein includes fish, meat, poultry, seafood, cheese, and eggs.

Women need about as much as the size of a deck of cards, men a bit more.

Breakfast tunes your body to lose weight. Eat breakfast every morning. The odds are better that you'll be at your ideal size soon.

Since you're following point 1 and 2 above and not eating toast or boxed breakfast cereal, here are some suggestions for breakfast:

- An egg and an apple or other piece of fruit

- 2 ounces cheese and fruit or vegetable

- Meat, fish, or poultry—even leftovers—with vegetables and fruit

- Small bowl of steel-cut oats, cooked, with an egg and fruit

- Small bowl of steel-cut oats, cooked, with 1–2 ounces of cheese and fruit

- For additional ideas, refer to the breakfast menus in appendix D of this book

If it's sour, devour it. Fall in love with acidic-tasting foods and eat them often, even at every meal. See the list in Chapter 4.

Add a big squeeze of lemon to your tea, and learn to prefer vinegar-and-oil salad dressings. Keep dill pickles, horseradish, and other vinegary condiments in the refrigerator and use them with vegetables and meats.

Don't sweat the small stuff. A spoon of sugar in your iced tea, the breading on a fish served at a restaurant, two or three corn chips with salsa before dinner, or one spoonful of rice with your stir fry is fine.

Eating the small stuff once or twice a day won't prevent weight loss; eating them more possibly could. But eating while you're preparing a meal is not small stuff—it's fattening. Don't do it.

If it contains gobs of fat, don't eat it. Don't get too strict with yourself about fat, unless you need to for medical reasons, but be mindful of eating too much. Eat these seldom, if at all: bacon, sausage, ribs, fried chicken, fried fish, french fries, and other high-fat foods. Check the labels on processed foods and dairy to make sure they aren't too high in fat.

Always eat 0–5. Eat only when you're hungry and stop eating when your stomach is comfortable, before you're full.

For beverages, drink purified water and herbal teas. You can consume a cup or two of caffeinated beverages such as tea and coffee every day. Late-afternoon lattes would count as one cup of caffeine—order them up with whole milk or skim milk.

As you read through the Keep It Simple plan, you'll see that it's really easy to dine out and eat with family and friends.

The only time we've been stumped for what to eat on the Keep It Simple program is when traveling abroad. We supplement the traditional continental breakfast of croissant and coffee with serving-size store-bought containers of tuna and some dried fruit that we packed along.

Yes, you can live well, healthy, and happily without eating starches, or by eating very few. Your body doesn't require them for nutrition. On the Keep It Simple program, eat starches selectively. If you have a favorite starch food, such as donuts or chocolate cake, you can have a normal-size piece of them occasionally. Be sure you don't eat a starch food you don't really love. In other words, don't eat that tempting slice of breakfast toast. Instead, carefully eat a starch that appeals to you most.

> **Body of Knowledge** _____
>
> Three to four ounces of meat, seafood, or poultry contains about 21 to 28 grams of protein. Three ounces is about the size of a deck of cards or the size of a small can of tuna. That's all the protein an average-size woman needs to eat three times a day to stay healthy. An average-size man needs to eat four ounces of protein three times a day. In other words, forget about ordering the 16-ounce rib eye at the steak house … unless you plan to feed four or five people!

Fine Tuning

As you begin the Keep It Simple program, check your body size or your weight only once every week. If you haven't seen a difference after two weeks, you may need to make one or more of the following adjustments:

- ◆ Take a careful and unbiased look at the amount of food you're eating and make your serving sizes smaller.

- ◆ Reread the nine points and make sure you're following them in fact and in spirit.

- ◆ Choose a low- to medium–glycemic treat instead of one that's high glycemic.

- ◆ Reduce your stress levels. See Chapter 23.

If these changes don't work, start keeping a detailed food diary and you will probably figure out what's not working. It's easy to get a bit sloppy when one doesn't keep notes. But one of the beauties of the Keep It Simple program is that you don't need to keep notes.

Foods to Eat Sparingly

As you eat the Keep It Simple way, here's a list of foods to avoid or eat sparingly:

- ◆ High-glycemic foods.

- ◆ Fruit juices. Eat fruit instead. The glycemic index and the glycemic load of fruit is lower than juice because the fiber in the fruit slows digestion and fruit contains a lower density of calories and carbohydrates. If you want juice, you can mix juice with water in the ratio of about ⅓ juice to ⅔ water and have one glass two or three times a week, preferably with a meal.

◆ Diet sodas. Aspartame and other artificial sweeteners. Some research shows they stimulate appetite. New research indicates they cause metabolic syndrome and lead to type 2 diabetes. Aspartame is in diet sodas and many other diet products. It's also used as a sweetener in yogurt and processed puddings and custards.

◆ Coffee and caffeine. Don't drink over two servings a day. If you love your morning coffee or tea, eat breakfast while you savor your "wake-up" brew.

◆ Alcoholic beverages. Limit yourself to one to two drinks a week. Alcoholic beverages can stimulate appetite, so they could derail your weight-loss efforts. But not everyone reacts the same way.

◆ Soft drinks and sodas. These are sticky foods. Instead drink water or herbal teas. If you crave flavor in your water, add a slice of lemon, lime, or orange. Or add the contents of one Emergen-C to water. Emergen-C in packets is widely available at health-food stores and grocery stores.

◆ Any food to which you're allergic or sensitive.

Eating these foods can stall your weight loss or lead to weight-loss plateaus. If you reach a plateau, start keeping a daily food journal. Most likely, you'll figure out what you're doing wrong.

The Comprehensive Program

The Comprehensive glycemic index weight-loss program incorporates all the details and nuances of the glycemic index. Choose the Comprehensive program if you …

◆ Want to or need to keep detailed eating records.

◆ Have an analytical mind and value precision.

◆ Have available time and energy to add up your food intake based on glycemic load.

◆ Can make modifications to your program based on your rate of weight loss.

◆ Need and like the structure that the Comprehensive program offers.

$\bigcap \bigcap \bigcap$ **-couragement** _____

To determine the glycemic load of your foods, you don't need a sharp pencil and calculator, but rather a good glycemic index list. Lists online at www.glycemicindex.com and www.mendosa.com now include the glycemic load for average serving sizes. You can use the list in Appendix B at the back of this book, too.

How Much to Eat

In the Comprehensive program, you'll be keeping track of your glycemic load. To start, you need to keep track of your food intake. Use this chart.

Glycemic Food or Beverage	Glycemic Amount	Index	Total Load	Time by Meal
_____	_____	_____	_____	_____
_____	_____	_____	_____	_____
_____	_____	_____	_____	_____
_____	_____	_____	_____	_____
_____	_____	_____	_____	_____
_____	_____	_____	_____	_____
Totals by Day _____		Glycemic Load Units _____		

Your goal is to eat 60 to 75 glycemic load units a day. You'll be eating about 15 to 20 each for breakfast, lunch, and dinner. An extra 15 to 20 are for snacks during the day. You can have two or three snacks per day.

Wrong Weigh _____

Don't save up glycemic load units or carbohydrate grams and then eat them all at one meal. This defeats the purpose of glycemic index weight loss. If you do this, you'll send your blood sugar and insulin levels soaring and your body will be inclined to respond by storing fat rather than by releasing it.

You'll need a notebook in which to keep your daily tally sheets. Plus, you'll need a good and reliable glycemic index, glycemic load chart, and carbohydrate gram chart. You can download the glycemic index with glycemic load from www.mendosa.com. The site has computer software you can order, too. With GlycoLoad, from www.phelpsteam.com/glycoload, your computer automatically calculates the glycemic load of any amount of food as long as you know how many ounces you plan to eat. You can also use the glycemic index and glycemic load listing in Appendix B of this book. And, you can use the list in the book *What Makes My Blood Glucose Go Up … and Down* by Jennie Brand-Miller.

What to Eat

On the Comprehensive program, you'll limit high-glycemic carbohydrates to less than 15 percent of your carbohydrate intake every day. Eat mostly low-glycemic carbohydrates or "free foods" and perhaps some medium-glycemic foods.

Your meals will look like this:

◆ At each meal, fill half of your plate with nonstarchy vegetables. For breakfast, you can substitute one fruit for a vegetable provided that the glycemic load for each meal is 25 or less.

◆ Eat about three to four ounces of animal protein. This is about the size of a deck of cards or a small can of tuna. Choose from meats, seafood, poultry, and eggs. Men can eat four ounces.

◆ You can eat breads, crackers, and pastas made with stone-ground or coarse-ground grains, and so on; just be sure that they're low glycemic. Cook pasta al dente, about 5 to 6 minutes and no longer. When you can, eat genuine stone-ground breads. Ditto that for crackers and muffins.

◆ Include dairy products, such as milk, yogurt, and cheese, keeping within your daily glycemic load recommendations. Plain yogurt and milk contain between 12 and 17 grams of carbohydrates per serving and have glycemic loads of about 2 to 4. One serving is one cup. Cheese has a 0 glycemic load and is mainly protein, so use it as part of your total protein food allotment. Eat no more than 1 ounce of cheese a day.

◆ Dessert can be a low-glycemic food, such as premium ice cream or fruit. Remember, though, to keep your food intake within 15 to 20 glycemic load units for each meal if you're eating a total of 60 to 75 glycemic load units per day.

Snacks can include stone-ground whole grain crackers with cheese, dried fruit, and vegetables and fruit. You can also choose snacks from the nonstarchy veggies list.

Read commercial bread labels carefully. If they contain caramel coloring, wheat flour, white flour, or dough tenderizers, they're most likely high glycemic. Instead, choose a bread that has just a few ingredients: stone-ground flour, yeast, salt, water.

$\displaystyle \mathsf{THIN}$ -couragement

> If you want to accelerate your weight loss, increase the amount of fiber you eat up to 45 grams per day. You can also add more acidic foods to your meals, as a way to lower the effective glycemic load.
>
> When computing the glycemic load of a meal, you can reduce the count by one third if you eat at least four teaspoons of vinegar in your salad dressing.

Monitoring Your Progress

On the Comprehensive glycemic index weight-loss program, you may need to adjust your total glycemic load for the day. If you find that after eating 60 to 75 glycemic load units a day for two weeks or so you aren't losing weight, you'll need to lower your glycemic load units. If you are counting carbohydrate grams instead of glycemic load units, you can lower your carb grams to as little as 15 per meal instead of 30 per meal.

You can lower the glycemic load unit amount to 50 or even 40, but we don't recommend going lower than 40 per day. Eating below 40 would put you in starvation mode and you're your metabolism. Continue to balance the load throughout the day. So if you choose to eat 50 units, divide them as follows: 10 to 15 for each meal and 5 to 15 for snacks.

Weight-Loss Expectations

Basically, there's no way to predict how fast you'll lose weight. Some factors that could make a difference are …

♦ **Age.** A general rule of thumb is that it takes longer to lose weight when a person is older because metabolism slows with age.

♦ **Current weight.** If you have lots of weight to lose, your initial weight loss could be faster than a person who only has 15 to 20 pounds to lose.

♦ **Metabolic rate.** If your body fat percentage is high, it could take longer than if it's low. If you have been told that you're metabolically resistant to weight loss, increase your strength-training exercise to lower body fat percentage and boost metabolism. Be sure to check out other factors in Chapter 6.

♦ **Food sensitivities and allergies.** Avoid eating these foods to speed up your weight loss. Common food allergies include wheat, gluten, soy, and dairy.

If you want to speed up your weight loss, be sure to read through this book and follow the suggestions to boost your metabolism, reduce stress, and use the power of your mind.

Body of Knowledge

If you suspect that you have food allergies or food sensitivities, set up an appointment with an allergist to test for possible food allergies. You can also avoid eating that food for a week and if your symptoms are gone, then try to cut that food out of your diet. But if you suspect that you are sensitive to more than one food, consulting with an allergist can help you unravel your body's reactions.

Don't be afraid of losing weight too fast with glycemic index weight loss. The meals you're eating are balanced, nutritious, and wholesome, so there's no danger that you'll be starving yourself.

Maintaining Your Weight Loss

The good news is that you can easily maintain your weight loss by continuing to eat based on the glycemic index. You'll keep doing what you're doing right now, but your food intake will be more liberal.

◆ On the Keep It Simple maintenance program, you can add one serving of low-glycemic grain-based food such as bread, rice, or pasta, if you don't have celiac disease or allergies to gluten or wheat. Try this for two weeks. If you continue to lose weight, add one more servings of a food you enjoy, being sure to continue to eat 0–5.

◆ On the Comprehensive maintenance program, you'll increase your glycemic load units by 20 for two weeks. If you're still losing weight, increase by 20 until you have stopped losing weight. Continue to balance the glycemic load among all three meals and snacks.

Keep your food portions the same for meats, seafood, and poultry—about three to four ounces per meal. You'll never need to eat more than this amount. Continue to fill half your plate at each meal with nonstarchy vegetables.

The Least You Need to Know

◆ You can choose between the Keep It Simple or the Comprehensive program for glycemic index weight loss.

◆ Eat two to three servings of nonstarchy vegetables or fruit at each meal.

◆ Eat mostly low-glycemic carbohydrates and only rarely eat high-glycemic ones.

◆ The maintenance programs are a relaxed version of the program you have chosen.

Part 3

Nutritionally Balanced Eating

Your glycemic index meal-planning is centered around eating moderate amounts of meats, seafood, poultry, and eggs along with 5 to 10 servings of vegetables and fruits every day. You can include stone-ground breads, whole grains, and low-glycemic cereals.

Make wise choices of lean animal protein and good fats. Learn how to incorporate dairy into your meals and find ways to enjoy sweet tastes without reverting to white sugars, white flours, and junk foods.

Supplement your food intake with nutritional and dietary supplements that give you support for glycemic index weight loss. Investigate supplements that enhance your digestion, plus those that soothe moods, balance your body's acid/alkalinity, and balance your electrolytes.

Chapter 11

Protein

In This Chapter

- ◆ Understanding the importance of proteins
- ◆ Using proper serving sizes
- ◆ Eating as a vegetarian
- ◆ Stocking your pantry

Perhaps you've tried one of those popular diet programs that urges you to eat as much meat and fat as you desire. Breakfast could have been ½ pound of fried bacon and four or even six eggs, and the results were promising—you could lose some weight. But you weren't eating healthfully. In fact, you could have been doing your body as much harm as good.

Things have definitely changed in the world of weight loss. You don't need to rush out to the grocery store to purchase massively huge sirloin steaks, rashers of bacon, and mountains of ground beef to lose weight. Instead, dine on moderate amounts of succulent meats, seafood, poultry, and eggs.

In this chapter, you learn how much protein and which kinds of protein your body requires to lose weight and maintain good health plus a high metabolism.

Your Body Needs Protein

When a person is accustomed to eating high-glycemic foods, protein becomes an afterthought. You might center your meals around pastas, breads, or potatoes. Or, like many of us, around what we thought was the only reason for eating a meal—the dessert.

What a mistake! Meals aren't supposed to be about indulging a sweet (or starch) tooth, but about eating important nutrients that support your health and well-being. We know now that one of the reasons people become overweight is because they missed that point.

The point is that each meal needs to include high-quality *complete protein*. Your body needs protein daily, and preferably three times a day. That's how you receive the all-important essential *amino acids* that are the building blocks of your body. They build muscle. They boost metabolism. They keep your hair, skin, and fingernails lustrous and glowing.

Glyco Lingo

Complete protein is protein that contains adequate amounts of all nine essential amino acids. Only animal proteins, such as meats, seafood, eggs, and dairy, provide this.

Amino acids are the chemical units that form proteins. They make up the muscles, ligaments, tendons, organs, glands, nails, hair, and even vital body fluids. They also help regulate all bodily and metabolic processes. The body needs to obtain nine essential amino acids through food regularly for good health.

And here's more:

- Proteins make up muscles, ligaments, tendons, organs, glands, nails, and hair, and are essential for strong bones.

- Proteins help regulate the body's water balance and maintain the proper internal pH balance. A lack of protein causes water retention.

- Proteins form the structural basis of DNA.

- Without adequate protein, the strength of your immune system is jeopardized.

- Proteins in the form of amino acids activate vitamin and mineral utilization by the body.

- Eating the right amount of protein assists your body in losing weight and maintaining weight loss.

- Proteins rebuild and restore body tissue and muscle.

- Eating protein slows down the digestion of sugars and starches and helps prevent a rapid rise in blood sugar levels.

As you can see from the previous list, you don't want to skimp on eating proteins. Instead, make sure that you eat some animal protein at every meal.

The Nine Essential Amino Acids

Only by eating high-quality protein can you obtain the nine essential amino acids found in food that are essential to bodily functions. The other 20 or so amino acids your body needs are manufactured in the liver by using the nine essential amino acids as the raw materials. Without the essential nine, your body simply won't perform properly.

Eating protein is vital to the liver's health and function. Fasting has been promoted as a way to lose weight and detoxify the body, but not eating enough protein actually prevents the liver from detoxifying. Fasting has never been shown to be a healthful or effective means for long-term weight loss.

Soy products offer you essential amino acids, but not at optimal levels. Soy is limited in methionine and tryptophan. Healthwise, small amounts of soy might be okay, but large consumption of soy products has been linked to thyroid malfunction and dementia. Soy products, such as roasted soybeans, tofu, and tempeh, are wholesome foods and can be eaten three to four times a week. Soy products need to be counted both as protein and as carbohydrates. You'll learn more about soy in Chapter 14.

Wrong Weigh

Because some egg substitutes and containers of egg whites contain additives, you may want to avoid any form of eggs that come as liquid. Go totally natural and crack your own.

Types of Animal Proteins

For your glycemic index weight-loss program, eat animal protein at least three times a day. Animal protein with the exception of some dairy products doesn't contain carbohydrates, so its glycemic index is zero with zero glycemic load. You can savor the following animal proteins:

◆ **Meats.** Beef, pork, buffalo, lamb, veal, and wild game such as venison, moose, and elk.

◆ **Poultry.** Chicken, turkey, duck, and Cornish game hens, along with wild game such as pheasant, quail, geese, duck, and doves.

◆ **Seafood.** Shellfish such as crab, shrimp, lobster, calamari, mussels, and clams, plus all fish found in oceans, streams, and lakes. This includes salmon, sardines, trout, bass, tuna, snapper, and the list goes on and on.

◆ **Eggs.** Eat the entire egg; both yolk and white contain protein. Research now indicates that eating only egg whites may not be beneficial to your health.

◆ **Dairy.** The only dairy product that contains virtually no carbohydrates is regular hard cheese, such as cheddar, Edam, feta, and Swiss. Cottage cheese and feta cheese contain about 6 grams of carbohydrates per cup. Low-fat cheeses, including low-fat cottage cheese, contain about 8 grams of carbohydrates per cup. Unsweetened dairy products have a low-glycemic index. Milk and yogurt offer you some protein, but not as much as other animal protein sources. Don't use milk or yogurt as your primary source of protein for a meal.

Vegetable Proteins

Soy products contain protein, as do many other vegetables. All legumes and nuts contain a significant amount of protein, and soybeans are legumes, as are peanuts. But when you're eating the glycemic index way, vegetable protein also counts as carbohydrates. The glycemic index of vegetable proteins, such as legumes, is low—usually ranging between 14 and 25.

Vegetable proteins are not complete proteins; they're *incomplete proteins.* They don't give your body all the power it needs in the realm of protein, and often vegetable protein is difficult for humans to digest and assimilate.

Vegetarians sometimes use food combining as a way to obtain adequate amounts of essential amino acids

> **Glyco Lingo**
>
> **Incomplete proteins** are foods that don't contain all nine essential amino acids in optimal quantities. These foods are vegetables or vegetable-based, such as soybeans, nuts, legumes, and grains.

from vegetables. They combine a legume with a grain, such as red beans and rice or corn and beans.

Food combining doesn't work well for glycemic index weight loss. By the time a person eats enough "brown rice and beans" to provide 15 to 20 grams of complete protein, the glycemic load would be off the acceptable chart for that meal.

Wrong Weigh

If you want to substitute cottage cheese for meat and fish, use these guidelines. An ounce of meat or fish is equivalent in protein to ¼ cup cottage cheese.

Serving Sizes

Your body's need for complete protein depends on the size of your frame and your activity level. Don't worry, there's no need for challenging calculations here. We make it simple.

Men need about 4 to 5 ounces of animal protein three times a day. Women need about 3 to 4 ounces. For women, that's an amount equal to the size of a deck of cards or a small can of tuna. Men need as much animal protein as 1½ decks of cards.

If a person orders a 16-ounce rib-eye steak for dinner, that's enough protein to feed four adults.

You don't need to eat more than the recommended amount. In fact, it's best if you don't overdo it. Overeating anything causes increased insulin levels, and it's now been found that eating too much protein over a long period of time can lead to insulin resistance. Some animal proteins also contain a significant amount of fat, and too much fat causes more insulin resistance. When a person is insulin-resistant, weight loss becomes more difficult.

THIN-couragement

It's a common misconception that eating the low-glycemic way is more expensive than eating a high-carbohydrate and high-glycemic all-purpose diet. But if you sharpen your pencil and calculate the difference between eggs and fruit versus cereal, milk, and juice for breakfast, the costs are just about equal. And if you include all the money spent on junk foods, sodas, and candy machines, low-glycemic eating may cost you less.

When you eat protein, the body releases small amounts of insulin, but not nearly the same amount as when you eat carbohydrates. When people eat excessive amounts of animal protein, however, not only do they increase their fat intake, but their insulin can rise far enough to affect fat storage. As you are learning, making sure you eat the right amount of each type of food is important for ultimate weight-loss success.

Vegetarian Choices

Being a vegan—a person who eats absolutely no animal products—and eating for glycemic index weight loss is very challenging. First of all be sure that you are a vegetarian—meaning you eat more vegetables, and not a "starcharian," meaning you eat lots more grains and starches.

Vegetarians who eat some animal products: eggs, dairy, cheese, and perhaps seafood, will find that glycemic index weight loss can work very well. Eat these forms of protein three times a day, making sure to eat 15 to 20 grams of protein and keep your glycemic load low. That's 3 to 4 ounces three times a day for women, and 4 to 5 ounces three times a day for men.

Unfortunately, it's easy to gain weight eating as a vegetarian. Often people will eat very small amounts of animal protein or none at all and, in its place, often because they develop food cravings, eat lots of starches. In effect, they've become "starcharians." The net effect is that they keep on gaining weight and losing muscle mass—and end up wondering why such an "inspired" way of eating is making them fat.

Low-glycemic eating is also an inspired way of eating, because it is in alignment with what the body needs to eat for health and proper body-sizing.

Selecting Animal Proteins

As you browse through the meat section of the grocery store, here's what to look for when selecting your protein entrées:

◆ If the seafood is fresh and smells mild, it's a good buy. Avoid fish that's been frozen and thawed, because it has lost flavor and needs to be eaten by the next day.

◆ Stock up on canned or vacuum-packed tuna, sardines, and salmon. These are caught wild and usually processed on ship or right off the ship. Use these for quick meals and snacks. Pack some along when you travel—just in case you can't find protein selections for breakfast or lunch.

- Shop wisely for price. Buy on sale when the store has a "buy one, get one free" promotion. Meat freezes well.

- Keep some frozen hamburger and chicken on hand for the times when you need to whip up a quick meal and you don't want to go to the store.

- Purchase lean meats. Trim all visible fat from meats before cooking. This reduces the total amount of saturated fat that you and your family will eat.

- Keep fresh, whole eggs on hand. They'll keep in the refrigerator for several weeks, but most likely, you'll eat them before then. Make boiled eggs so they're handy for snacks or quick meals. They're great to add to tuna-fish salad.

- Many grocery stores offer a wide selection of cheeses from around the world. Find some you particularly enjoy and eat for snacks and meals.

- Purchase sliced meats—turkey, roast beef, or ham—at the deli and use for lettuce wraps, luncheon salads, and breakfast omelets. Be sure to ask for all-natural meats.

Be sure to keep plenty of protein in your refrigerator, freezer, and pantry so you always have something to eat for meals and snacks.

THIN-couragement

New research shows that eating whole eggs for breakfast helps women lose weight and have more sustained energy. It only takes about 3 minutes to cook an egg for breakfast in a small amount of butter or olive oil.

The Meat Controversy

Perhaps you've read or heard about the antibiotics and growth hormones added into the feed of livestock. To say the least, it's controversial. No one is sure of the long-term health effects of eating meat raised with these additives.

If you are concerned, purchase "drug free" meats. They are more expensive, but you may feel that the extra cost is well worth it.

Another controversial aspect about livestock is its diet. Most livestock are corn fed. Researchers have found that corn-fed beef is higher in saturated fat and lower in omega-3 essential fatty acids than grass-fed beef. Grass-fed beef is available at natural-food grocery stores and, like the drug-free beef, it costs a little more than grain-fed beef.

Farm-raised salmon contains toxins and contaminants such as polychlorinated biphenyls (PCBs). Additionally, the fish is treated with coloring before being sent to market to make the flesh appear pinkish-red. Farm-raised salmon naturally has a gray color. If you want to avoid eating farm-raised fish, you can purchase wild salmon at stores. Canned salmon and sardines are generally caught in the wild and are either processed on the boat or at the canneries on the coasts.

The Least You Need to Know

- Eating moderate amounts of complete protein is essential for your health and for successful glycemic index weight loss.

- Only animal protein contains all nine essential amino acids in adequate amounts and is recommended for low-glycemic weight loss.

- Eating as a vegan is highly challenging with glycemic index weight loss. If you are a vegetarian, you can more easily eat low glycemic.

- Keep your kitchen stocked with a wide variety of animal proteins.

Chapter 12

Dietary Fats

In This Chapter

- ◆ Eating enough fat
- ◆ Avoiding fat-induced insulin resistance
- ◆ Enjoying the benefits of fat for glycemic index weight loss
- ◆ Understanding the importance of essential fatty acids

The word *fat* itself seems fattening. As recently as 10 years ago, some health experts advocated eating only 5 to 10 percent fat in one's daily food intake. Popularly accepted thinking was that eating fat made a person fat, as if it went directly from mouth to thighs and waistline. That thinking is wrong.

Perhaps you followed a low-fat diet for a while and stocked your kitchen with many of the low-fat margarines and salad dressings. If you haven't done so already, you'll be tossing some of these out and visiting the grocery store to purchase some full-fatted products. You'll be shopping for the good fats, such as omega-3s and monounsaturated fats. These types of fats in the right amounts can provide health and weight loss.

Eating the right fats helps you lose weight on a glycemic index weight-loss plan. In this chapter, you learn all about your body's need for fat, which specific types of fat are beneficial for you to eat, and which ones you should avoid.

The Fat-Insulin Resistance Connection

Eating fats is important for losing weight. But eating fat can also be detrimental, depending upon how much and what types of fat you eat. Some types of fats can actually cause insulin resistance. Also, eating too much fat—over 40 percent of your calories from fat—can cause insulin resistance. The bottom line on fats is that some is good for you, too much is bad for you, and too little is also bad for you.

Reducing or eliminating your body's insulin resistance is one of the significant reasons to eat the glycemic index way, so you certainly don't want the types of fat or the amount of fat you eat to lead you back to yet more insulin resistance.

Studies show that two types of fat—saturated fats and trans-fats—cause more insulin resistance compared to other fats.

Saturated Fats

Saturated fats are found in whole and low-fat dairy products such as cream, milk, half-and-half, butter, cheese, and ice cream. Saturated fats are also found in meats such as beef, pork, poultry, and lamb.

Your body can handle some saturated fats just fine. About 10 percent of your food intake can be saturated fat. When you consistently eat more than that amount, insulin resistance can arise. You can also become insulin-resistant if you eat more than 35 percent of your daily calories from fat. A high intake of saturated fats is also linked to heart disease.

Trans-Fatty Acids

Trans fats are not natural. They were created in the laboratory by modifying cooking oils to increase shelf life. Trans fats are bad for your health. They've been shown to directly cause heart disease and other chronic health conditions.

The FDA now requires that food manufacturers list the amount of trans fats per serving on food labels. If the label reads 0 trans fats, the serving could contain up to

0.5 gm based on FDA regulations. Read the serving size carefully. Some food processors make the recommended serving size very small so they can claim 0 trans fats per serving. A small bag of chips may suggest 3 servings, which, if you ate all the chips, could make the total trans fats you eat 1.5 grams.

Trans fats are present in processed and prepared foods, such as cookies, breads, frozen foods, and crackers. Margarines, solid vegetable fats, and homogenized peanut butters also contain trans fats.

Food manufacturers are finding ways to eliminate trans fats from food. But some restaurants are not finding it easy. Trans fats are used for frying foods, such as french fries and chicken. But as of this writing, few fast-food restaurants have found acceptable substitutes for trans fats. So you have one more good reason to avoid french fries—in addition to being high glycemic, they contain trans fats.

Good Fats Are Good for You

Eating fat helps you lose weight—that is, when you eat the right amount and types. Your body needs monounsaturated fats and polyunsaturated fats, which can include the healthy essential fatty acids.

Monounsaturated Fats

Nutritionists recommend that 10 percent of your daily food intake come from monounsaturated fats. Health benefits of monounsaturated fats include:

- They help reduce insulin resistance.

- They lower blood levels of LDL, the "bad cholesterol," without affecting levels of "good cholesterol," HDL.

- They are chemically stable fats and may help in protecting against certain cancers, such as breast cancer and colon cancer.

- They help support the immune system.

Wrong Weigh

Just because a fat such as olive oil is good for you doesn't mean that more is better. You only need to eat about 4 tablespoons of fat or oil a day based on a food intake of 1,500 calories. Enjoy the olive oil, but don't pour it on; instead, drizzle it on.

- They don't produce inflammatory prostaglandins in the body like some fats, so they are protective and help with inflammatory conditions such as rheumatoid arthritis, dementia, diabetes, and heart disease.

- In the right amount, they help you lose weight.

Monounsaturated fatty acids, also called omega-9s, are present in larger quantities in the following foods:

- Almonds
- Avocados
- Brazil nuts
- Cashews
- Hazelnuts

- Olive oil
- Olives
- Peanut oil
- Peanuts
- Sesame seeds

These foods either contain no carbohydrates or are low glycemic. The vegetables and nuts listed above are high in dietary fiber, except for olives.

Polyunsaturated Fats

Eating 10 percent of your daily food intake from *polyunsaturated fats* is important. There are two types: omega-3 and omega-6 *essential fatty acids*. They're very important for your health and weight loss.

Glyco Lingo

Polyunsaturated fats are dietary fats that aren't "saturated." They're liquid at room temperature and remain liquid when refrigerated or frozen.

Essential fatty acids (EFAs) are polyunsaturated fats that you need to eat every day. Your body can't manufacture them from other foods, hence the government designation "essential." The two main essential fatty acids are alpha-linolenic acid (an omega-3 fatty acid) and linoleic acid (an omega-6 fatty acid).

Omega-3s and omega-6s need to be eaten in the correct balance. In our modern diet, it's easy to eat plenty of omega-6 fats, but not so easy to eat enough omega-3 fats. Ideally, the balance is one part omega-6s to two parts omega-3s.

Eating Omega-3 Fats

Alpha-linolenic acid (ALA) is metabolized in the body and converted to eicosapentae-noic acid (EPA) and docosahexaenoic acid (DHA). EFA and DHA are found only in cold-water fish. They're important for weight loss, heart health, aids to mood disorders, anxiety, and depression. Add to that shiny and radiant hair, nails, muscle tone, and healthy joints and skin.

While some people synthesize EPA and DHA from alpha-linolenic acid, some people don't. That's why everyone is advised to obtain EPA and DHA directly from fish and fish oil.

Here are natural sources of omega-3 fatty acids:

◆ Alpha-linolenic acid (ALA)—cold-water fish and fish oils, flax seeds, and flaxseed oil

◆ Eicosapentaenoic acid (EPA)—cold-water fish such as ocean-going salmon, herring, tuna, and cod

◆ Docosahexaenoic acid (DHA)—cold-water fish, some algae

Following are some of the benefits you'll enjoy from omega-3 essential fatty acids:

◆ They facilitate brain neurotransmitters so that they lift moods, reduce anxiety and depression, and stabilize bipolar disorders.

◆ They support your immune system.

◆ They reduce inflammation throughout the body, including in joints and skin.

◆ They help soothe allergic reactions.

◆ They assist releasing unneeded stored fat.

◆ They improve heart health by lowering cholesterol and triglyceride levels.

◆ They help reduce facial wrinkles and sagging.

Wrong Weigh

Some people's bodies aren't efficient at converting alpha-linolenic acid into EPA and DHA. That's why it's best to eat cold-water fish or take fish oil capsules or liquid to consume EPA and DHA directly. Cold-water fish include salmon, cod, tuna, and herring.

On your glycemic index weight-loss plan, eat cold-water fish to make sure you receive the full weight-loss and health benefits of these amazing fatty acids. Eat three to four servings a week. You can also take fish oil supplements. You learn more about supplements in Chapter 16.

Eating Omega-6 Fats

Omega-6s are more common in today's diet, and you probably consume more than you need. The omega-6s contain the essential fatty acid linoleic acid, which is found in raw seeds and nuts and corn, and sunflower, cottonseed, safflower, and soybean oils.

The omega-6 fatty acids are valuable, especially the gamma-linolenic acids. GLA helps protect against inflammatory conditions such as rheumatoid arthritis, diabetes, and heart disease, to help with nerve transmission, eczema, psoriasis, premenstrual syndrome, and benign breast disease.

Omega-6 foods that are high in gamma-linolenic acid include …

- ◆ Borage oil, found in health-food stores.

- ◆ Black currant oil, found in health-food stores.

THIN**-couragement**

Your daily fat intake needs to be about 20 to 35 percent of your total food intake divided as follows: one third, or about 10 percent each, of monounsaturated fats, polyunsaturated fats, and saturated fats.

Food sources of omega-6s with lower amounts of GLA include …

- ◆ Soybean oil.

- ◆ Pumpkin seeds and pumpkin seed oil.

- ◆ Sunflower seeds and sunflower seed oil.

- ◆ Safflower oil.

- ◆ Corn oil.

Omega-6 food sources include butter, palm kernel oil, coconut oil, and red meat.

The Least You Need to Know

- ◆ Overeating fat in general, and overeating saturated fats or trans fats, can increase insulin resistance.

- ◆ Low-fat processed foods may contain high-glycemic carbohydrates.

- ◆ Avoid eating trans fats, also known as hydrogenated and partially hydrogenated vegetable oils.

- ◆ Eat fish that contains essential fatty acids at least twice a week or take a tablespoon of fish oil daily to help you lose weight and boost health.

Dairy

In This Chapter

- ◆ Discovering dairy's uniqueness
- ◆ Eating dairy's many varieties
- ◆ Counting dairy carbohydrates
- ◆ Dealing with dairy sensitivity

Some of us just love dairy products. They have been part of our daily diets since childhood, basically from birth! We drank milk as children, we spooned it up with our breakfast cereals, and we all screamed for ice cream. The ice cream man jangled through our childhood neighborhoods on hot summer afternoons, and probably still does so.

Dairy products are unique as natural food products. Dairy is the only food that contains significant amounts of the basics: animal protein, saturated fats, and carbohydrates. (Hard cheeses, though, contain very few, if any, carbs.)

For someone on a glycemic index weight-loss program, dairy foods can be tricky. Dairy can be included in your diet, but if you're sensitive or allergic to dairy, you need to avoid it. In this chapter, you learn the complexities of dairy products and how to include dairy in your glycemic index weight-loss program.

The Animal Connection

Dairy is unique as a food. It's not easily categorized. Dairy comes from animals and contains substantial healthful protein. In its natural form, it contains plenty of saturated fat, although you can reduce the fat by using low-fat and nonfat versions. Some dairy foods are moderately high in carbohydrates, although some dairy foods have few carbs. When left unsweetened, dairy products are low glycemic. Unsweetened dairy products include plain milk, cream, some cheeses, and yogurt.

THIN-couragement

> Most low-fat processed foods have added high-glycemic fillers that can make them off-limits for low-glycemic eaters. But this isn't true for all low-fat dairy products. You might need to be more careful with the lower-fat sweetened dairy, since many of these products can be too high in refined carbohydrate and, consequently, have a higher glycemic load.

Here's the dairy nutritional scoreboard. Note that the different types of dairy products offer quite different amounts of carbohydrates and saturated fats. All nutrition counts are given in grams.

The dairy nutritional scoreboard includes some surprises. As you can see, one cup of milk contains 12 grams of carbohydrates, almost as many carb grams as a typical slice of bread. Plain or unsweetened yogurt contains between 12 and 16 grams of carbohydrates. The biggest difference is that milk and yogurt are low-glycemic foods with a glycemic load of 3 to 4, whereas white and whole-wheat bread are high-glycemic foods with a glycemic load of 9 to 10.

Body of Knowledge

> Although butter clearly comes from the milk of a cow, it's not considered a dairy product from a nutritional point of view. Instead, butter is categorized as a fat. It contains saturated fat, but no carbohydrates. It's fine to use small amounts of butter, being sure to keep your intake of saturated fat to 10 percent or less of your total fat intake.

Dairy Product	Amount	Carbs	GI (Glycemic Index)	GL (Glycemic Load)	Protein	Saturated Fat
Whole milk	1 cup	12	31	4	8	8
2% milk	1 cup	13	32	4	8	5
Skim milk	1 cup	13	32	4	9	0
Cream	2 TB.	1	0	0	0	9
Half-and-half	2 TB.	1	n/a	n/a	1	3
Cottage cheese 4%	½ cup	3	n/a	n/a	13	5
Cottage cheese 2%	½ cup	4	n/a	n/a	13	3
Cottage cheese (nonfat)	½ cup	5	n/a	n/a	13	0
Hard cheese	1 oz.	0	0	0	6	10
Low-fat cheese	1 oz.	1	0	0	8	4.5
Cream cheese	2 TB.	1	0	0	4	20
Cream cheese (light)	2 TB.	2	0	0	3	4.5
Cream cheese (fat-free)	2 TB.	2	0	0	10	0
Whole yogurt (unsweetened)	1 cup	12	36	3	9	10
Yogurt light (unsweetened)	1 cup	16	36	3	10	4
Yogurt (fat-free, unsweetened)	1 cup	16	36	3	10	0
Ice cream (full-fat or premium)	½ cup	17	38	5	3	9
Ice cream (light)	½ cup	19	50	5	3	4.5
Ice cream (fat-free)	½ cup	22	47	5	3	0

High in Saturated Fats

In Chapter 12, you learned that saturated fats need to be eaten in moderation, with preferably only 10 percent of your daily food intake coming from saturated fats. Eating high amounts of saturated fats can increase insulin resistance, the very thing you want your glycemic index weight-loss program to prevent or correct. One way to reduce the amount of saturated fat in dairy is to consume mostly fat-free dairy products or low-fat versions.

Glyco Lingo

CLA (conjugated linolenic acid) is thought to be helpful in weight loss by promoting the use of stored fat for energy.

Some high-fat dairy products such as butter, cheese, and premium ice cream are good sources of *CLA (conjugated linolenic acid)*. In some studies, CLA has been shown to reduce body fat mass. Don't overeat high-fat dairy products, but consume them within a balanced diet.

Dairy and Weight Loss

Should you eat dairy products if you're on a glycemic index weight-loss program? Some research studies show that consuming dairy products while on a restricted-calorie diet speeds up weight loss and reduces body fat percentage. Some researchers think that the calcium in dairy might be the reason. And, indeed, studies show that the calcium in dairy products seems to promote weight loss. However, new studies show that calcium in any form helps with weight loss, not just dairy.

If you prefer not to eat dairy products or you are allergic to dairy, however, other forms of calcium can help you lose weight. You can get calcium from salmon and sardines, seafood, dark-green leafy vegetables, almonds, asparagus, cabbage, figs, hazelnuts, and calcium supplements.

Be sure that you include milk as a food in your daily food journal. Some clients were at a weight-loss plateau and yet consumed three glasses of milk daily. They weren't factoring the milk into their total food intake!

Calcium is best absorbed in the body when vitamin D, magnesium, vitamin C, vitamin A, some trace minerals, and a sufficient amount of high-quality protein are present. But too much phosphorus, sodium, caffeine, wheat bran, protein, and alcohol can decrease the absorption of calcium.

Calcium absorption is also aided by doing moderate levels of exercise, as you'll be doing on your glycemic index weight-loss program.

Body of Knowledge _____

Calcium is an important nutrient for more than weight loss. Calcium builds strong bones and teeth and keeps gums healthy. Calcium helps prevent cardiovascular disease by lowering cholesterol levels and blood pressure levels. Calcium aids in brain neurotransmitter regulation and the prevention of muscle cramps. In addition, calcium appears to reduce the risk of colon cancer by binding bile acids and free fatty acids in the colon.

Dairy Sensitivities and Allergies

Dairy is great if you can tolerate it. Perhaps you're one of the many people who don't do well with dairy products. If you experience the following symptoms after eating dairy, it's best to avoid them:

- Bloated feeling
- Gas or flatulence
- Phlegm in your throat or head
- Clearing your throat frequently
- Constipation
- Diarrhea

With these kinds of symptoms, you could have a food sensitivity or food allergy to dairy or to the sugar present in milk and yogurt, lactose. Whenever you experience such symptoms, make a record of what foods you ate that may have caused the symptoms. That way, you can pinpoint the offending food.

Food allergies can cause mucus buildup throughout the body and within the digestive system. Bloating, gas, and excess phlegm are symptoms of your body's protective reaction to the allergens. Alas, this buildup of mucus also causes weight gain. When you stop eating the offending food, the mucus buildup dissolves, is excreted, and your weight returns to normal.

An allergy to dairy is different from intolerance to dairy products. Most milk intolerances are due to being lactose intolerant. Dairy allergies are associated with reacting to the proteins in the dairy products.

If you have lactose intolerance, you may be able to tolerate dairy by taking a lactase enzyme dietary supplement when eating dairy products. If this works for you, great. If not, don't despair. Many people who can't tolerate high-lactose dairy products such as milk and yogurt can tolerate lower-lactose dairy products such as cottage cheese and hard cheeses. If you can't tolerate dairy, you can still consume calcium in other forms.

Here are other foods that deliver calcium without dairy:

- Dark-leaf green vegetables, such as kale and spinach.

- Salmon and sardines, with the bones. Canned are great!

- Asparagus, broccoli, cabbage, and other green vegetables.

- Nuts and seeds, such as almonds, filberts, sesame seeds, and flax seeds.

- Calcium dietary supplements. Take one that breaks down easily and contains magnesium.

THIN**-couragement**

To determine whether your calcium supplement breaks down easily for digestion, put the calcium supplement in a glass with 6 ounces of cider vinegar. Stir every 5 minutes. If the tablet or capsule dissolves within 30 minutes, it will dissolve in your stomach.

The 5 to 10 servings of vegetables and fruits that you're eating daily plus complete protein three times a day provide many of the nutrients that are needed for calcium absorption.

A Healthful Concern

The dairy industry has come under attack in recent years. Dairy products may contain antibiotics, bovine growth hormone, and other drugs used to enhance milk production. The FDA allows these chemicals to be used in milk production, but questions remain as to their ultimate long-term safety.

If this concerns you, buy organic milk and milk products that are available in health-food stores and in many regular grocery stores.

The Least You Need to Know

- Dairy is the only food group that contains animal protein, saturated fat, and carbohydrates.

- Some dairy products, such as milk, yogurt, and ice cream, can be high in carbs, whereas others, such as hard cheeses, are low carb.

- The calcium in dairy products and other foods helps you lose weight and keep it off.

- If you are sensitive or allergic to dairy, use alternative food sources of calcium plus calcium supplements.

14

Soy

In This Chapter

- ◆ Getting to know soy
- ◆ Varying versions of soy
- ◆ Determining low-glycemic soy foods
- ◆ Learning the health factors of soy

In this chapter, you learn about the different types of soy-based products, how they stack up on the glycemic index, and if they can deliver glycemic index weight loss. You also learn what the latest research studies have found about the long-term use of soy-based products.

A Thoroughly Modern Food

Soy products have been touted as an excellent diet food, and many popular diet programs recommend drinking their brand of soy shakes once or twice a day. Most soy shakes are low in fat and have a fair amount of soy protein isolate, *but* the protein has a low *biological value (BV)*. It sounds as if the soy shakes are great … but.

Although soy was revered as one of the five sacred crops in China over 5,000 years ago, its vast popularity has soared only in the past 30 to 40 years in the United States. Until recently, people, mostly Asians, ate soy primarily as a green legume, as edamame, or fermented in products such as tofu, natto, tempeh, miso soup, and soy sauce.

Glyco Lingo

Biological value or **BV** is a measure of how much nitrogen from the protein is absorbed, retained, and used by the body. Nitrogen is the key element in protein. BV determine how much protein the body can actually digest and assimilate from the food. A higher BV means better absorption. A whole egg is 100, soy is 74.

These fermented forms of soy are the most easily digested and assimilated. The fermentation process makes the proteins and other nutrients in soy more bioavailable.

One common misconception about soy is that it was and is a mainstay of the diet for Asian peoples. It wasn't, except perhaps for the poor and underprivileged people or in times of famine. Otherwise, they ate small amounts of soy products, but mostly focused their diets on foods with higher nutritional value: fish, meat, and vegetables.

After World War II, however, the whole nature of soy as a food and agricultural product changed. It became a significant part of agribusiness in the United States. Soy provides an inexpensive source of vegetable protein. It's low in fat and high in some of the essential amino acids, although not all of them.

Soy contains smaller amounts of *methionine* and *tryptophan*, two of the nine essential amino acids. Soy has a relatively low biological value (BV) of only 74, whereas whey protein has a BV of 104 and a whole egg has a BV of 100. Cow's milk is 91 and beef is 80. Don't plan on using soy-protein products to meet all of your daily protein needs. They can't.

In the past 30 years, the number of soy-based products has increased dramatically. You can drink soymilk, eat toasted soy nuts, and add soy-protein isolate to your baked goods. Soy shakes are easy to prepare. Just add water to a powdered mix. Soy-based protein bars sit alongside the candy bars at grocery stores and fast-food counters.

Doctors and food manufacturers often recommend soy formulas for infants and soy shakes for oldsters. Vegetarians use soy-based products as a meat substitute. Nutritionists credit the phytoestrogens in soy as beneficial for relieving menopausal hot flashes and discomforts.

Glyco Lingo _____

Methionine is one of the nine essential amino acids. It's also a powerful antioxidant that neutralizes hydroxyl radicals—one of the most damaging kinds of free radicals. Methionine assists in the breakdown of fats, helps digestion, and plays a role in maintaining muscle tone. As you can see, methionine helps you reach some of your weight-loss goals.

Tryptophan is a precursor to serotonin in the body. Serotonin is the brain neurotransmitter responsible for feelings of being soothed and uplifted. Many prescription antidepressants help increase amounts of serotonin in the brain. Tryptophan plays a role in manufacturing niacin, one of the B vitamins, and it plays a role in the repair of tissues.

Glycemic Index of Soy

Soy is classified as a legume—a bean. The basic soybean is low glycemic, as are most of the foods derived from soy. Following is a sampling of the GI of some soy-based products:

> Toasted soy nuts: 18
>
> Boiled soybeans or edamame: 18
>
> Soy infant formula: 55
>
> Soymilk: Ranges from 32 to 44
>
> Soy yogurt: 50
>
> Canned soybeans: 14

Tofu hasn't been tested, so for now consider it low glycemic and in the range of 10 to 20.

Tempeh hasn't been tested, so as with tofu, consider it low glycemic, at about 10 to 20. *Soy protein isolate* hasn't been tested, but you can estimate it's also in the 10 to 20 range.

Glyco Lingo _____

Soy protein isolate is a white powder derived from soybeans through a manufacturing process. This process isolates the protein from other components of the soybean. Soy protein isolate is added to many foods and is a popular ingredient in protein shakes.

Following is a sampling of the GI of a medium-glycemic, soy-based product and a high-glycemic product:

Medium-Glycemic:

Soy protein shake mixes that also contain modified food starch, corn syrup solids, sweet whey, maltodextrin, or sugar.

Soymilks with the previously mentioned additives.

Soy protein energy bars with high-fructose corn syrup, maltodextrin, sugar, or modified food starch.

Power bars: 56

High-Glycemic:

Soy protein products that contain food flavor mixes with additives such as those stated previously.

Tofutti frozen dessert: 115

If sugar or modified food starch is added to a soy-based product, the glycemic index value rises, as you can tell with the medium-glycemic power bars and the very high-glycemic Tofutti.

In addition to the additives listed here, many processed soy products also contain partially hydrogenated oils (trans fats), which aren't healthy to eat. Be sure to read the labels and the serving size to determine how much trans fat is in your favorite bars. You may want to switch to one that is both low glycemic and trans fat free. The USDA recommendation is to have no more than 2 g of trans fat per day, if any at all.

By reviewing the glycemic index information, it seems like soy is great for your glycemic index weight-loss program. But let's look further at some product characteristics and scientific research.

Limitations

Soy has limitations and strong critics as well as strong supporters. Soy products have become controversial because research points to health concerns about eating large quantities of soy-based products. Before you decide how many servings you want to eat per week, you need to learn about the concerns and decide for yourself.

◆ Soy has a low biological value, BV, compared to other protein sources, and it doesn't contain all nine essential amino acids in optimal quantities. To obtain a higher-quality complete protein you need to add animal protein such as meats, eggs, dairy, poultry, whey protein, or fish to your meals.

◆ Most soy products are processed foods, some more than others. Only green soybean, edamame, whole soybeans, and soy sprouts could be considered unprocessed natural "whole" foods. Soy protein isolate is highly processed as are soy milk and soy formula. Fermented products such as tempeh, natto, and miso are not as processed and the culturing of these products improves the bioavailability of their protein and other nutrients. The isolated protein powders are comparable to other highly processed foods, such as enriched white wheat flour and white sugar, because they're far removed from their natural state. Processed soy-based products contain very little, if any, dietary fiber.

THIN-couragement

Whey protein powder comes from milk and contains all nine essential amino acids in optimal amounts and has a high biological value of 104. You can add whey powder to your soy shakes or you can make shakes with whey powder alone.

◆ Many people have food sensitivities or allergies to soy. After eating soy, they feel bloated and gassy. These people aren't able to attain adequate digestion and assimilation of soy. If you have this reaction, stop eating soy products.

◆ Soy contains protease inhibitors that make it difficult for your body to break down amino acids. Also, soy contains high levels of phytates and oxalic acid that interfere with the absorption of many nutrients. Protease inhibitors, together with phytates and high levels of oxalic acid, can impair your immune system.

◆ In the concentrated soy-based products, such as tofu, soymilk, and soy protein isolate, the phytoestrogens content is also concentrated. Some menopausal women experience symptom relief with soy products, but the amount of phytoestrogens consumed may not always be consistent, and because of this, some members of the medical community feel it is not a reliable way to help with hot flashes.

◆ The concentrated protein and isoflavones in soy-based products can depress thyroid functioning and lead to hypothyroidism. This slows metabolism and makes it harder to lose weight. If you eat lots of soy and you've been diagnosed with an underfunctioning thyroid, stop soy for a month. You may find that you can stop your thyroid medication. Be sure to consult with your medical practitioner.

- Long-term studies of people who eat soy-based products show an increased risk of dementia later in life.

- Soymilk baby formula may be related to attention deficit disorder, learning disabilities, and behavioral problems in many children.

The final word on the safety of soy hasn't been written. To say the least, however, soy is controversial. If you'd prefer to avoid the controversy altogether, don't eat or drink soy-based products. If you love soy, eat it wisely, as described next.

Eating Soy

You can overeat any kind of food. Certainly it's easier to overeat treat foods, such as chocolate, donuts, and chips. But there's also another kind of overeating. It comes from thinking that if a little of one food is good for one's health, more of it is better.

This isn't the case with soy. A little can be good for you; more can possibly be harmful. Our suggestion is, if you are not sensitive to soy, have one serving one to four times a week, and no more. Make soy a small part of your diet and not the main course. If you choose to eat soy, choose the easiest to digest and more nutritious soy products such as edamame, tempeh, natto, or miso.

From a nutritional point of view, it's best to eat a wide variety of foods and to avoid eating any food repeatedly. Yes, even chocolate.

The Least You Need to Know

- Soy-based ingredients are present in over two thirds of all manufactured foods.

- Soy-based products, such as tofu, soymilk, and soy protein isolate, are highly processed forms of soybeans.

- Soy has a low biological value and contains limited amounts of two essential amino acids, methionine and tryptophan.

- Negative health studies on soy make it a controversial food that needs to be eaten infrequently, if at all.

Chapter 15

Sugars and Junk Foods

In This Chapter

- Identifying junk foods

- Limiting sugar

- Avoiding artificial sweeteners

- Reading ingredient lists

- Shopping for low-glycemic treat foods

Just about everyone loves junk food. This has to be true. Otherwise, grocery stores wouldn't devote so much valuable shelf space to fulfilling our country's overwhelming preference for these products.

Look on any high-traffic corner in any city or town in the United States. What do you see? Fast-food establishments that dish up millions of high-glycemic, junk-food meals daily.

We all know these foods are only marginally acceptable for sustaining life and that they offer little, if any, nutritional value or health benefits. Yet junk-food eating goes on and on. Avoiding non-nutritious empty foods can be difficult and exasperating, and it seems that junk food is here to stay. But it doesn't need to stay in your kitchen.

In this chapter, you learn about sugars and the junk ingredients to avoid. As a conscientious consumer of low-glycemic foods, you also need to beware of products that claim to be beneficial to your diet. Many packaged low-carb, low-sugar foods can fool you and aren't the slightest bit good for your weight or your health and aren't necessarily low glycemic.

The Low-Glycemic Health Concept

Low-glycemic weight-loss programs are specifically designed for you to lose weight. That's their first and primary purpose, and that's why you're reading this book. But the secondary benefit of glycemic index weight-loss is that you can become healthier in general.

As you release stored fat, you naturally reduce the risk or reality of heart disease, high blood pressure, and diabetes. You're also becoming naturally healthier for the long term because you're eating very nutritious foods. As you continue to eat lean meats, good fats, and plenty of vegetables, your body begins to feel great. You have more energy, your skin glows, and overall, eating is simple because you use a clear plan.

The glycemic index weight-loss program highly recommends that you continue eating healthful foods. But plenty of "bad-for-you" foods are often more widely available than the "good-for-you" foods. Here's what you need to know to enjoy the good and avoid the bad. The statements in this list are blanket statements, and you will find exceptions to all of them. But generally speaking, these are what you should avoid:

- If the packaging is a fun color and very cute, what's inside is junk food.

- If the food or beverage has an unnatural color, such as cotton candy, bubble gum, or a blue or chartreuse-colored sports drink, it's junk food.

- If the food is in the middle aisles of the grocery store, on the end caps, or at eye level, it's most likely junk food—high in carbs, sugar, or fat. This isn't always true, so check the ingredient list.

- If the food looks like a candy bar, but claims to be a nutrition bar, it could be junk food. And it's probably high glycemic, but not always.

- If your children beg you to buy it for them, most likely it's junk food. We have never met a child yet who begged for string beans.

- If it's for sale in a gas station or convenience store, consider it junk food. Only rarely can you find even an apple in a roadside stop.

Read the label to be sure it doesn't contain more than two or three *mystery ingredients.* If you want to eat healthy, you should totally avoid eating foods that contain more than two or three mystery ingredients.

Glyco Lingo

Mystery ingredients are food package ingredients that you can't pronounce, are ingredients that you can't actually purchase by themselves at the grocery store (such as maltodextrins), or are preservatives and artificial colorings or flavorings. Avoid purchasing products with more than two or three mystery ingredients, if any.

Sugar, Plus Variations

To tell the honest truth without any bias toward what's healthful, sugar simply tastes wonderful. In a sense, it doesn't actually taste like anything other than utter sweetness. Sugar has a mystery all its own. Part of the mystery is its overwhelming allure; part is how something that tastes so divine can be so bad for us. It doesn't seem fair.

Now that nutritionists and health-food gurus know the downside of sugar, many millions of research dollars have been poured into finding a sweet-tasting substitute. Ideally, the substitute would be better than neutral for your health—it would actually be good for you. So far, those millions haven't found the sweet fountain of great taste and great health. The search continues.

Any sweetener, whether natural or artificial, is thought to cause a beta-endorphin increase in your body that stimulates sugar cravings, so it's best to use all sweeteners sparingly. But until the time when a really great substitute is created or discovered, here's the lowdown on available sweeteners:

◆ **Table sugar, or sucrose.** Surprise! Sugar isn't high glycemic. It's medium. But who eats sugar all by itself? Add it to flour and the combination usually becomes high glycemic—think cakes and cookies. Just 1 teaspoon contains 4 grams of carbohydrates, 15 calories, a glycemic index of 61, and a glycemic load of 2.5. Sugar is acceptable in small amounts if eaten infrequently and as part of a balanced meal.

◆ **Natural cane sugar.** This is tricky labeling language for sugar, sometimes sprayed with brown coloring. It has the same stats as table sugar. There's not much special about it except the name.

- **Brown sugar.** This is also sucrose sprayed with brown coloring. It has the same stats as table sugar. Usually brown sugar is a darker brown color than natural cane sugar.

- **Evaporated cane syrup.** This ingredient appears on labels for foods that are sold at health-food stores. Beware. This is simply another fancy and healthy-sounding name for table sugar, also known as sucrose.

- **Fructose.** The sugar found in fruits and honey. Good for you when eaten in fruits and honey. Not so good when overeaten. This could mean eating too much fruit at one time, drinking a large glass of fruit juice, drinking or eating foods sweetened with high-fructose corn syrup, or using too much packaged fructose crystals as a sweetener in foods. Just 1 teaspoon has 4 grams of carbohydrates, 15 calories, a glycemic index of 19, and a glycemic load of 1.

- **High-fructose corn syrup.** A highly controversial product used in too many processed foods, including sodas, electrolyte beverages, baked goods, and candy. It's made from genetically modified corn. A teaspoon contains 5 grams of carbohydrates and 20 calories; the glycemic index and glycemic load are unavailable. Avoid this product. It has been shown to raise triglyceride levels, which lead to heart disease and weight gain.

- **Agave nectar.** Made from agave cactus. Available at health-food stores. A teaspoon contains 5 grams carbs, 16 calories, a glycemic index of 10, and a glycemic load of 1.

- **Honey.** Naturally occurring—even the caveman and cavewoman ate honey. It's the only true paleo-sweetener. But obtaining honey in those days was a tricky and challenging endeavor, so it was probably eaten infrequently. A teaspoon contains 6 grams of carbs, 20 calories, a glycemic index of 55, and a glycemic load of 3. Honey gives you some unique nutritional benefits. It can be helpful for people who suffer from seasonal allergies, and it contains small amounts of minerals and B vitamins.

THIN**-couragement**

If you have seasonal airborne allergies and would like to use bee products for nutritional support, use bee pollen rather than honey. Bee pollen has virtually no carbohydrates but plenty of B vitamins. Take a very small amount at first, as it can cause an allergic reaction. If bee pollen suits you, you can take up to one teaspoon a day.

◆ **Other syrups, such as molasses, rice syrup and barley syrup.** Contain carbohydrates and calories similar to corn syrup.

◆ **Aspartame.** Also known as Equal, is a widely used artificial sweetener. Aspartame is non-nutritive and is GRAS—generally recognized as safe—by the FDA. It's an ingredient in diet sodas and thousands of other processed foods, such as sugarless yogurt, popsicles, and lemonade. Some research studies conducted since FDA approval indicate that aspartame may not be safe or good for weight loss. Aspartame is now known to increase the risk of metabolic syndrome and cause weight gain. It also increases beta-endorphin production, which triggers sweet cravings. Because its safety is in question and a vigorous controversy continues to grow, we can't recommend aspartame. Aspartame will stall your weight-loss program.

◆ **Sucralose.** Also known as Splenda, is another artificial sweetener. It's derived through chemically altering table sugar by adding chlorine molecules. Sucralose is 600 times sweeter than table sugar and doesn't raise blood sugar and insulin levels. The FDA has approved it as GRAS (generally recognized as safe) as a sugar substitute, but, as in the case of aspartame, some new research indicates that long-term use could present health problems. Many people like sucralose, but we can't wholeheartedly recommend it.

◆ **Stevia with FOSs.** It is not an artificial sweetener, but rather a totally natural product. Stevia is an herb from South America that's safe and without side effects. It's 300 times sweeter than sugar. When combined with FOSs—*fruit ogliosaccharides*—it has a smoother taste and is 10 times sweeter than sugar. It's widely available at grocery stores and health-food stores. We highly recommend stevia with FOSs as a sweetener. Its glycemic index is 0. Just ¼ teaspoon, which is very sweet, has less than 1 gram of carbohydrates and zero glycemic index value. You can also use plain stevia as a sweetener, if you like. Major soft drink manufacturers have announced they'll be using Stevia as a sweetener soon.

> **Glyco Lingo**
>
> **Fruit ogliosaccharides (FOSs)** are a probiotic nutritional supplement that selectively nourishes the friendly bacteria in the intestines. This increases the number of good bacteria in your gut. Not only is stevia safe, FOSs are definitely good for you.

◆ **Sugar alcohols.** Also called polyols. Some, such as mannitol, are used in making sugarless candy. Don't be fooled. Sugar alcohols still have calories. They don't increase blood sugar levels as much as sugar, because they are incompletely absorbed into the bloodstream. Chemically, sugar alcohols aren't sugar, so food manufacturers can claim their products are sugar free. One big drawback is that eating too much of them can cause flatulence and diarrhea.

It is important to note that sugar alcohols increase blood sugar, but not to the same high level as high-glycemic foods. The American Diabetes Association adds sugar alcohol counts to carb counting when the food contains more than 10 grams of sugar alcohol per serving. For foods that contain more than 10 grams, they count ½ of the sugar alcohol grams as part of the total carbohydrate count for the meal.

Common sugar alcohols include mannitol, sorbitol, xylitol, lactitol, isomalt, maltitol, and hydrogenated starch hydrolysates. Mannitol, sorbitol, and xylitol occur naturally in fruits and vegetables.

Unlike other sugar alcohols, xylitol can offer some health benefits because it isn't fermented by oral bacteria, so it doesn't cause tooth decay, and xylitol inhibits bacterial growth.

Junk-Food Ingredients

Food processors and manufacturers want to create foods that people will want to eat. These are foods that taste so good that people are compelled to purchase them over and over again. In essence, they're selling calories, and the population as a whole loves high-carbohydrate calories wrapped in exciting packaging with fun colors that contain virtually no nutritional value.

But what's in the package or what's not in the package makes a difference to your weight-loss success. So here's a list of ingredients you want to avoid.

◆ **White flour.** Also known as enriched flour, made from whole grains, fortified, and sometimes labeled natural. Instead, choose products that list whole-grain unrefined flours and grains.

◆ **Fruit drinks.** Usually sweetened with high-fructose corn syrup or other sugars, such as evaporated cane sugar. These are filled with sugar and offer very little real fruit value. They're definitely not one of your 5 to 10 servings of vegetables and fruit for the day.

- **Fruit juice.** A highly concentrated form of fruit without any of the beneficial dietary fiber. You're better off eating real fruit. Check the label, and if it's pure juice with no additives, it's medium glycemic and okay to have once in a while. You can dilute fruit juice with an equal amount of water for a less sweet-tasting drink.

- **Food starch.** Fillers such as maltodextrins and modified food starches are high glycemic and high in calories. They're used to add bulk to food, just like they do to you.

- **Partially hydrogenated vegetable oil or hydrogenated oils.** These are trans fats, which should always be avoided. Even eating a few grams a day is thought to increase the risk of heart disease.

- **Artificial coloring.** A non-nutritive chemical that only adds color, and could cause a reaction in some sensitive individuals.

- **Preservatives.** Used to extend product shelf life, and not considered healthy.

- **Monosodium glutamate, or MSG.** Used as a flavor enhancer, it actually mimics the taste of proteins, which is why it's often added to foods such as soups, bouillon, and packaged meat products. MSG is known to cause headaches and discomfort in some people.

- **Olestra.** Used as a fat substitute and can cause upset stomach. Many food manufacturers are no longer using this product because of undesirable side effects.

- **Foods fried in trans fats.** At this writing, many fried foods are still fried in partially hydrogenated vegetable oils also known as trans fats. This includes french fries and onion rings, as well as fried chicken and fish fillets. Many restaurants and fast-food chains are now frying foods in oils without trans fats. Be sure to ask before you order.

- **Dough tenderizers and other odd ingredients.** If it simply doesn't make sense to you, pass on it.

You can usually find some high-quality packaged food items at health-food stores and in some grocery stores in the health-food section. However, continue to read labels, because even totally organic foods can be junk foods. Organic lemonade sweetened with organic evaporated cane syrup is junk food. Organic evaporated cane syrup is another way of saying table sugar.

The Low-Carb Shelf

Grocery stores are stocking more and more low-carb processed foods as consumers continue to realize the benefits of eating the low-carb way. But beware! Low carb doesn't necessarily mean low glycemic, or that you're eating a healthy food.

You need to read the ingredients. Look for foods that contain few preservatives and no high-glycemic ingredients, such as enriched wheat, modified food starch, high-fructose corn syrup or artificial sweeteners. Also, make sure the ingredients are every-day foods, and not such things as modified food starches and partially hydrogenated vegetable oils. The best place to find high-quality and highly nutritive low-glycemic foods is on the outside perimeter of the grocery store. There you'll find vegetables, fruit, meats, and fish. You absolutely can't go wrong eating the basic foods of glycemic index weight loss.

The Least You Need to Know

- ◆ Eating junk foods is not compatible with eating for glycemic index weight loss.

- ◆ Eating healthful, nutrient-dense foods ensures your weight-loss success and boosts your health.

- ◆ Use sugars and sweeteners sparingly to prevent cravings and avoid nutritionally devoid carbohydrates.

- ◆ Carefully read packaged food labels and avoid eating the ones with too many mystery ingredients.

Chapter 16

Nutritional Supplementation

In This Chapter

- ◆ Improving your digestion and assimilation
- ◆ Unwinding stress with B vitamins
- ◆ Using minerals to manage insulin resistance
- ◆ Keeping your electrolytes balanced

Taking one-a-day or two-a-day or maybe even more-a-day vitamins and supplements can make glycemic index weight loss happen faster. When your body is missing or is low on some important nutrients, your weight-loss efforts can stall.

That's not to say that simply by taking the right mix of nutritional supplements you can lose all the weight without reducing your food intake. That won't happen. But combining the two may prove to be a great solution. Eating the glycemic way and using nutritional supplements that support your body together will help you release stored fat. In fact, you can make up for lost or missing nutrients from when you were eating fewer healthful foods.

The Need for Supplements

Controversies about nutritional supplementation have raged for years. One side asserts that all the vitamins and minerals people need can be assimilated from the food they eat. The other side strongly suggests that, although that was once true in the good old days, it's no longer true today.

You know which side is winning. Just look up the number of health-food stores in your phone book or on the Internet, or visit the nutritional-supplement section of any grocery store, drugstore, or discount chain. People buy supplements and plenty of them.

In the good old days, fruits and vegetables were picked ripe and eaten within hours. Food animals grazed freely on grassy plains. Fish were caught fresh from streams, lakes, and oceans and eaten soon afterward. "Junk" was something people threw away, not something they ate joyously and eagerly. In short, during those good old days, food contained more nutritional value than it does today.

Wrong Weigh

Check out Internet sites that offer supplements before you purchase. Some offer low prices on brand-name products and offer handy reorder shopping carts. Beware the sites selling too-good-to-be-true weight-loss supplements. You'll find more hype than substance.

Obviously, you can live without taking nutritional supplements. But we don't know why you would want to. All evidence points to people living better and healthier lives with a little help from health-food stores. Health practitioners and doctors are now widely recommending that their patients take nutritional supplements.

Losing weight is challenging. And a little or even a lot of help along the way is available to you in health-food stores, drugstores, Internet sites, or discount chain stores.

In the United States, the FDA does not consistently enforce quality standards for dietary supplements. Supplement manufacturers aren't legally required to test their products to verify that they contain standard and consistent amounts of natural herbs, minerals, and vitamins. As a result, consumers may consume varying amounts of an herb or vitamin with each bottle they purchase. The products can also contain filler ingredients, which could cause allergic reactions in some people. Here are some guidelines to help you purchase safe and effective products:

- Buy only commercially sold products from reliable sources. The label should include a list of the ingredients in detail. Look for the GMP (Good Manufacturing Processes) stamp of approval. To have this stamp is optional, but it does mean that the company is inspected and goes through safe and reliable manufacturing methods and that it lists all ingredients on the label as well as the specific amounts of these ingredients.

◆ Buy standardized extracts whenever possible. This provides you with some assurance that the active ingredient is present in the amounts you want and expect.

◆ Purchase supplements and use them before the expiration date. Store all supplements in a cool, dry place. If the supplement requires refrigeration, be sure to refrigerate.

◆ Don't buy supplements that contain excessive doses of trace minerals. High doses of one mineral can offset the benefits of another. For example, too much zinc can interfere with the absorption of copper.

Following are some guidelines for optimizing the use of supplements:

◆ Take most supplements with or immediately after a meal. The digestive enzymes and hydrochloric acid secreted when you eat help break down not only the nutrients in the food, but also those in the supplements.

◆ Some supplements, such as some amino acids taken for a specific purpose, need to be taken on an empty stomach as indicated on the label.

◆ Take one new product at a time. If the product is causing adverse reactions, it can be easier to detect.

◆ Some natural remedies contain potent chemicals that can interfere with absorption or other medicines you might be taking. Talk to your pharmacist or doctor to check on drug-supplement interactions. You can often find this information online as well. Your need for specific supplements can change from time to time, so once or twice a year evaluate which supplements you're taking. Make changes if it seems necessary. If you take a lot of tablets or capsules, you may be able to consolidate some or possibly eliminate them from your daily regimen.

Your Digestion, Assimilation, and Elimination

The first place to start when you consider nutritional supplementation isn't with a vitamin pill. Instead, the place to start is with your body's digestion, assimilation, and elimination mechanisms. You can be taking the most expensive and powerful vitamin and mineral supplement in the world, but if your digestion and assimilation processes aren't working well, your body isn't going to realize the benefits.

THIN **-couragement** _____

It's easy to think that if you didn't digest your food well you'd lose weight easily. The body is more complicated than that. Before you'd lose weight, your body would think it was starving, utilize some muscle for fuel and conserve fat. You'd get flabby and your body fat percentage would increase. You'd even gain weight and have a tough time losing it because your body would hoard the excess fat.

Digestion is a very complicated process. To digest your food well, you need to have your digestive enzymes functioning well, and you need an adequate amount of hydrochloric acid to be present in your stomach. Very frequently, by the time a person reaches 35 to 40 years, digestion becomes less efficient. The person isn't receiving the full nutritional value of the foods he or she eats. Given that many foods people eat are already low in nutrients, such as junk foods, the body isn't receiving enough value from the foods eaten.

Body of Knowledge _____

A large number of people with cystic fibrosis, celiac disease, and Crohn's disease have an important need for pancreatic enzymes that their body does not make on its own. The rest of us can use digestive enzymes to aid our digestion. Symptoms of indigestion include bloating, belching, abdominal pain, excess gas, foul-smelling stools or stools that float, diarrhea, and constipation.

Digestive Enzymes

Stress causes havoc with efficient digestion. Stress blocks adequate production of digestive enzymes because it slows the parasympathetic nervous system. In addition, age decreases our ability to produce hydrochloric acid and digestive enzymes. Taking digestive enzyme supplements can be a boon if you're over the age of 35 to 40, and maybe for some younger people. Digestive enzymes may help your body receive nutritional value from the foods you eat, and they can help your body digest the nutritional supplements you take.

The signs of poor digestion are burping, bloating, constipation, diarrhea, gas, acid reflux, and irritable bowel. Long-term inability to digest some types of food can be found in weak nails, poor skin quality, dull or thinning hair, poor muscle tone, and lack of energy.

Individuals with indigestion could possibly benefit from taking a general all-purpose digestive enzyme supplement.

Look for the following components:

◆ Enzymes that digest protein include bromelain, pepsin, papain, and protease.

◆ Lipase is an enzyme that digests fat.

◆ An enzyme that digests carbohydrates will be useful now that you're eating complex carbs such as vegetables and whole grains. The enzymes that digest carbs are amylase or invertase.

Many digestive enzyme products available at the store work to digest all three: proteins, fats, and carbohydrates. Try one. Then, if for any reason you don't like the results, select a different brand or formulation until you find the one that works best with your body. Most products on the market are not that potent and will not cause a lot of problems if you don't need them; however, don't take excessive doses of digestive enzymes, it may result in gastrointestinal adverse effects, such as nausea, vomiting, diarrhea, and abdominal cramps. So take what's suggested on the label and take only with food. If you don't experience a change in your digestion after taking them for a couple of weeks, you can discontinue them.

Elimination

It's impossible to lose weight if you don't have a bowel movement daily. It only makes sense that to eliminate weight you need to eliminate. Do everything you need to do to make this happen. Some clients seldom have a bowel movement and are very frustrated that they can't lose weight. If constipation is a serious problem for you, consult with your health practitioner. Here are some ways to promote good bowel activity and health:

◆ Don't eat foods to which you're allergic. They can cause diarrhea or constipation.

◆ Eat 25 to 45 grams of fiber daily. Supplement with additional fiber if needed, increasing slowly over a couple a weeks up to 25 grams. See fiber section that follows.

◆ Take good bacteria such as acidophilus daily, either through cultured milk products or a dietary supplement.

◆ Drink purified water—about 6 to 8 glasses daily.

◆ Make sure you don't have yeast overgrowth syndrome. You can clear yeast overgrowth by taking plenty of good bacteria. Keep your body alkaline by eating 3 servings of vegetables and fruit every meal, taking cream of tartar 2 to 3 times a day, and eating sour/acidic foods often. Consult with your health practitioner to find natural ways to yeast.

Wrong Weigh

We haven't known anyone who has had success in clearing yeast overgrowth syndrome by eating a yeast-free diet. Instead, look to ways to keep your body alkaline, because yeast can't overgrow in an alkaline body.

You can find other solutions for constipation at a health-food store and in reference materials such as books and the Internet. No single solution works well for everyone, so keep searching until you find what works for you.

Herbs

Herbs can be excellent digestives. Many old-fashioned desserts contained herbs to help settle the stomach. Think peppermint, black pepper, ginger, and fennel seed.

Specific herbs that help stimulate the secretion of digestive enzymes include gentian, bitter melon, dandelion, horehound, prickly ash, and artichoke.

Herbs have been used for centuries to relieve symptoms of indigestion, especially for excessive gas: anise, basil, caraway, cinnamon, cloves, fennel, dill, peppermint, sage, thyme, turmeric, and lemon balm. For heartburn, try teas of ginger, licorice, or slippery elm.

THIN-couragement

For a delicious digestive tea, steep 1 tsp. of fennel seeds in a cup of hot water. The seeds will settle to the bottom of the cup. Enjoy the sweet licorice taste as excess gas and stomach discomfort ease. Fennel and chamomile teas are sometimes recommended for colicky babies.

Fiber

By eating a low-glycemic diet, you'll automatically be getting a good amount of fiber; however, you may want to add a fiber supplement.

Body of Knowledge _____

Here are additional ways you can enhance the digestion and assimilation of nutrients: eat smaller portions at each meal. Eat in a relaxed atmosphere. Stress and eating on the run cause a decrease in your body's ability to secrete HCL and digestive enzymes. You can also eat a bitter or sour type of food or seasoning at the beginning of a meal. Examples of this include bitters, endive, lemon, limes, and vinegar. When you chew your food thoroughly and eat slowly, you also improve digestion and assimilation.

Fiber supports your entire digestive and assimilation function. Most people eat fewer than 15 grams of fiber a day. But you need 25 to 45 grams of dietary fiber every day to have regular elimination and increase food transit time through the body. You can't expect to lose weight if you aren't having at least daily bowel movements.

Fiber has other benefits:

◆ Fiber absorbs toxins and allergens from food and transports them quickly through the body.

◆ Fiber gives you a feeling of satiation when eating. Basically, fiber fills you up and the full feeling reduces your desire to overeat.

◆ Fiber slows the absorption of sugars and starches in the stomach, thus helping you avoid insulin resistance.

◆ Fiber helps reduce or eliminate both diarrhea and constipation.

◆ A high-fiber diet helps with some digestive disorders.

◆ Fiber helps lower blood cholesterol and triglyceride levels, and may also reduce the risk of developing gallstones.

THIN-couragement _____

Robin was 70 pounds overweight. She was only having one bowel movement every two to three weeks. No wonder she couldn't lose weight. Her body was holding on to everything she ate. Robin experienced painful backaches due to the backup of waste products in her bowels. Fortunately, fiber supplements worked for her, and her glycemic index weight-loss program began to work. As her elimination system began to function properly, she lost weight.

The easiest, healthiest, and least expensive way to take fiber is to consume psyllium. You can purchase psyllium in large bulk bags at health-food stores. It's unsweetened and unflavored, so it has no taste. Mix a heaping tablespoon of psyllium in a glass of water and drink quickly, before it starts to gel. Follow with another glass of water.

Each heaping tablespoon contains about 7 grams of fiber and no carbohydrates or calories.

Wrong Weigh

Avoid taking psyllium products that contain flavorings and sweeteners, whether the sweetener is sugar or artificial. You don't need the additives.

Good times to take psyllium are when you awaken before breakfast or just before bed. You can also take psyllium before or after a meal. Don't take fiber supplements at the same time you take medications or other nutritional supplements. The fiber could absorb them and diminish their effectiveness.

The Good Bacteria

Your digestive supplementation needs to include intestinal support for the good bacteria so that your body can efficiently assimilate the nutrients from your food. You need abundant amounts of good bacteria in your intestines. The good bacteria are wiped out when you take antibiotics, and it can be hard to repopulate them after you're finished taking the medication. Here's what the good bacteria does:

THIN-couragement

Good bacteria thrive on fruit ogliosaccharides (FOS), which are present in vegetables and fruits, as well as in the natural sweetener stevia with FOS. What a great reason to eat your veggies and enjoy the sweet taste of stevia with FOS.

- Produce some B vitamins. B vitamins are important for all bodily metabolic processes, and they also help reduce stress. Plenty of overeating is prompted by stress.

- Compete in the gastrointestinal tract with pathogenic organisms and protect us from harmful pathogenic by-products.

- Function as an antifungal. It helps reduce yeast overgrowth syndrome as well as other fungal infections.

- Enhance the absorption of nutrients.

If you don't have enough good bacteria in your intestines, you may experience gas, bloating, constipation, malabsorption of nutrients, and perhaps Candida overgrowth syndrome (also known as a yeast infection).

Good bacteria are acidophilus, lactobacillus, and bifidobacterium bacteria, plus some others. You can purchase them in pill, capsule, or powder form. Most brands need to be kept refrigerated. If you travel frequently or find it inconvenient to keep the supplements refrigerated, purchase a version that doesn't require refrigeration.

You can take the good bacteria supplements up to three times a day, apart from when you take fiber supplements. Take one to two capsules or tablets one to three times a day.

Now that your digestion, assimilation, and elimination are in good working order, it's time to start taking additional supplements for nutritional support.

) H||\\ **-couragement**

> In a study done by the University of Pretoria in South Africa, vitamin C helped combat stress by lowering cortisol levels by up to 30 percent.

Vitamins and Minerals

You need a vitamin and mineral supplement that contains all the basics including the following:

◆ **The B vitamins.** Some of these are the hardest to digest and assimilate, but now that your digestion is in tip-top shape, your body can benefit from taking B vitamins as a nutritional supplement. Because B vitamins are water soluble, unused portions are flushed from the body daily—so you need to replenish them daily.

B vitamins are used up quickly when you're stressed, and the mere fact of being on a weight-loss plan is stressful. And that's not counting what else is going on in your life. Take a B-vitamin formulation made specifically for high stress. Take one per day or follow the label guidelines, if different.

◆ **Vitamin C.** This vitamin is important as an antioxidant, and it's required for at least 300 metabolic functions in the body. Take up to 1,000 mg a day.

◆ **Vitamin E.** In its natural form, it helps balance hormones and helps prevent free-radical damage due to excess oxidation that can occur both with excess weight and during weight loss.

) H||\\ **-couragement**

> You can take liquid B vitamins sublingually, meaning under your tongue. This delivery method bypasses your stomach and digestive system entirely. Instead, the B vitamins are absorbed through the mucous membranes of your mouth. You can find liquid B vitamins at the health-food store. You can also use them when you feel highly stressed or need quick energy.

◆ **Vitamin D3.** Known as the sunshine vitamin. Your skin manufactures it when exposed to strong sunlight. Vitamin D helps your body utilize calcium, boosts your immune system, maintains healthy blood sugar levels, reduces osteoporosis, and helps protect you from diabetes, autoimmune disorders, and even cancer. If you live north of Atlanta, you probably don't have enough sunshine for your skin to make vitamin D. Take supplemental vitamin D3 in capsule form or take cod liver oil along with essential fatty acids.

◆ **Calcium.** Low calcium levels increase the stress hormone cortisol's ability to increase stress-related fat. Calcium helps burn fat by decreasing levels of lipoprotein lipase, a fat-storing enzyme. Several studies show that inadequate calcium in the diet is related to weight gain and that calcium aids in weight loss. The RDA (Recommended Daily Amount) for calcium is 1000 to 1300 mg. If you're a woman over age 35, make sure you take 1300 mg. You can take this separately from your vitamin/mineral supplement. A good combination is calcium with vitamin D3.

◆ **Magnesium.** Magnesium is depleted when a person has insulin resistance. Magnesium also helps the body use insulin effectively and safely. You also need magnesium to avoid muscle cramps and to soothe nerves. Take a magnesium supplement starting with 250 mg a day on up to 750 mg a day. Take magnesium to bowel tolerance, meaning until you get loose or runny bowels. If you develop diarrhea, cut back the amount of magnesium until your stools are normal. In general, the amount of magnesium you take should equal one half the amount of calcium you consume.

◆ **Chromium.** Assists the cells in uptaking insulin, so it aids you with eating the low-glycemic way and keeping your insulin levels balanced. Chromium helps build muscle, decrease body fat, and lower cholesterol levels. Take between 300 and 800 mcg per day. Start with a smaller dosage and increase it if you need more.

◆ **Vanadium.** Helps your body's cells absorb blood sugar more effectively, thus reducing insulin resistance. There is no RDA for vanadium, but nutritionists recommend you take between 40 and 100 mcg a day. Most people only require 40 mcg, but if you already have diabetes, you could benefit from taking more. If you prefer not to take a supplement, foods that are high in vanadium include black pepper, shellfish, parsley, and mushrooms.

◆ **Selenium.** Helps enhance the action of vitamin E as an antioxidant and is thought to help in the prevention of diabetes. Take 30 mcg a day.

Confirm that your vitamin/mineral supplements actually contain the ingredients listed on the label. Look for a UPS verified seal.

Some vitamin/mineral products are formulated specifically for persons who are diabetic, who have insulin resistance or metabolic syndrome, or who are eating the low-glycemic way. Check out those first before you purchase several bottles of supplements. It's obviously easier to take 1 or 2 capsules or tablets a day than to take 10 or 20. But overall, it's quite important to take the supplements you need for health and weight loss. If you're going to commit your energy to eating a low-glycemic diet, you want to give yourself every opportunity to succeed. The right supplements make it easier.

The Good Fats

Your body needs essential fatty acids (EFAs) every day, not just to facilitate weight loss but to also enable you to feel your best. These important fats actually let you release stored fat. But they do far more than that. EFAs keep your moods elevated and keep your joints and muscles in good working order.

Take from 1 teaspoon to 1 to 2 tablespoons of an essential fatty acid liquid once a day. This can be flaxseed oil or a combination of plant and animal oils. Or take 4 to 12 capsules of fish oil a day.

You can also eat cold-water fish, such as salmon, cod, herring, and sardines, three or more times a week in place of taking supplements. Or take the supplements *and* eat the cold-water fish. Just make sure you eat plenty of essential fatty acids.

If you prefer to take fish oil capsules and find that you burp the taste of fish oil, keep them frozen. Don't defrost, just take them frozen. The burps will be gone. Also, if you are on a blood thinner, talk with your health-care professional before taking fish oil.

THIN-couragement

The more you eat junk foods and highly processed foods that contain omega-6 polyunsaturated fats and partially hydrogenated vegetable oils (trans-fatty acids), the more omega-3 fatty acids you need to consume to keep your body in balance. But overall it's best not to eat junk food and factory-sourced food.

Helpful Supplements

In special circumstances, the following supplements are highly beneficial for weight loss. Whether you will need them depends on the state of your body and your health.

> ### Wrong Weigh
>
> If you have repeated or continual yeast infections, chances are good you find it impossible to lose weight. Most yeast infection remedies and diets are only marginally effective. A yeast-free diet is grueling and won't work if your body stays acidic. Try a greens drink. It can work within a week or two.

Electrolytes are great for cellular replenishment after exercise, sweating, or stress. They keep your body hydrated. Electrolytes are mineral complexes of potassium, magnesium, sodium, and calcium. Electrolytes can also give you a quick energy boost after a long day spent driving or sitting in meetings. Avoid using electrolyte beverages that contain sugars, high-fructose corn syrup, or artificial sweeteners. Instead, use electrolyte powders you mix with water. Our favorite brand is Emergen-C. You can find boxes of Emergen-C at health-food stores and grocery stores. It's great-tasting, and costs about 20 cents a packet.

"Greens" drinks are wonderful at killing off Candida and yeast overgrowth conditions. Yeast can't live in an alkaline environment. They thrive when your body's acid/alkaline balance is too acid. Greens drinks are actually powders made from all sorts of vegetables. You mix a tablespoon in a glass of water and drink it down. Usually 1 or 2 tablespoons a day are plenty to rid your body of a yeast overgrowth condition. Then simply drink a glass of greens several times during the week to keep your body in a slightly alkaline state, which will keep those yucky yeasties at bay. Overall, greens drinks are very healthy for you and provide you with many phytonutrients, antioxidants, vitamins, and minerals.

> ### Body of Knowledge
>
> Your body can become too acidic from incomplete digestion, eating high-glycemic foods, artificial or factory-sourced foods, taking prescription medications, or eating foods to which you are allergic. Allergic reactions to foods or the environment make the body acidic. Use suggestions in this chapter to correct your body's alkaline/acid balance.

When you feel your body needs a restorative tonic after travel, vacation, business meetings, or illness, try taking a greens drink for a couple days. Chances are good the tonic will refresh your body and rebalance your energy.

Supplements to Avoid

Beware of quirky supplements that promise you a simple, easy way to enjoy weight loss. Simple weight loss simply doesn't exist. Here's a list of some questionable products or ingredients that are currently highly promoted:

◆ **Bitter orange.** Bitter orange is extracted from Seville oranges, the ones from which orange marmalade is made. It sounds safe enough, and is in very small, naturally occurring quantities. But the extract is full of amphetamine-type stimulants that artificially boost your metabolism. You could lose weight and stored fat quickly. Then you'll experience the rebound effect and gain the weight all over again.

You probably remember bitter orange's cousin, ephedra, that's now banned in the United States by the FDA. Bitter orange, also known as citrus aurantium, is on the watch list of the FDA. They've had plenty of reports that it's not safe. Some commercially advertised weight-loss pills contain bitter orange. Pass on it.

◆ **Carb blockers.** These sound as if they would be wonderful. A person could eat a dozen donuts and not digest the carbs. This reasoning is flawed. Carb blockers are basically a form of dietary fiber that absorbs some of the sugar and starch from foods you eat and prevents them from being absorbed.

You could take carb blockers, but you can do just as well by eating foods high in fiber and using a fiber supplement such as psyllium. On a glycemic index weight-loss program, you are eating nutritionally important and healthy carbohydrates, so you don't need to block their absorption.

◆ **Fat blockers.** Fat blockers are marketed as weight-loss supplements that block fat absorption. They haven't been proven effective for long-term weight loss. The side effects, such as bowel leakage, are pretty disgusting. Pass on anything that could be this embarrassing.

Wrong Weigh

Fat blockers can't distinguish between fat from french fries and the good fats that are essential for your health. In addition, fat blockers decrease the absorption of fat-soluble vitamins such as vitamin E. You don't need to spend money on fat blockers. Instead, use the money to purchase good fat supplements and fresh vegetables.

If any other "miracle" weight-loss supplements come your way, check out the fine print.

The Least You Need to Know

- ◆ Put your digestion, assimilation, and elimination in tip-top working order to receive the utmost benefit from foods and supplements.
- ◆ Vitamins and minerals give your body support for blood sugar and insulin regulation as well as for weight loss.
- ◆ Use greens drinks to kill off yeast infections that otherwise can prevent weight loss.
- ◆ Avoid supplements that promise you'll lose weight.

Part 4

4

Eating for All Occasions

Eating at special events can be fun and delicious when you eat based on the glycemic index. You won't be afraid of parties, family get-togethers, and potlucks after you learn how to navigate the buffet table.

Grocery shopping requires that you learn new patterns and skills. Find out what aisles and sections to frequent and which ones to avoid. Cooking meals based on the glycemic index for yourself and the entire family can be easy when you remember to focus on "meats and vegetables" with flourishes, sauces, condiments, and variety.

Chapter 17

Eating a Meal or a Snack

In This Chapter

◆ Savoring low-glycemic foods

◆ Eating without stress

◆ Creating a soothing eating environment

◆ Appreciating snacks

Eating is a requirement of life. You need to eat. As you've figured out by now, there's no way you can avoid eating. You need to eat to survive, and if you're like most people, you need to eat at least three times a day and perhaps more, especially if you like to snack.

Fortunately for us, in addition to being a requirement, eating is highly pleasurable. Most of us like to eat. Food tastes good and appeals to our senses of sight, smell, and taste. We even stimulate our sense of touch when we eat with our fingers, handle food in the kitchen, and chew and swallow.

You already know how to eat, but do you know how to get the utmost pleasure from your food and the process of eating? You might find that as you derive more pleasure from eating, you are satisfied with less food. In this chapter, you learn the sensuous way to eat a meal or a snack so that all your senses feel satisfied.

Love the Food You're With

To use a line (modified for our purposes) from an old song, "If you can't be with the food you love, then love the food you're with." Adopting that attitude as you eat the low-glycemic way can make your meals a lot more fun. You'll find that it's easy to eat low-glycemic at most restaurants and social outings, as the basics of good eating are the same as the basics for glycemic index weight loss.

In the past, dieting and food restriction may have meant boring and unpleasant mealtimes. You may have found your food choices limited and unpalatable, or you may have watched the rest of your family members wolfing down the starchy foods you craved while you were left sitting with melba toast and a thin slice of cheese.

With glycemic index weight loss, mealtimes will change for the better. So start telling yourself that you love vegetables and salads. Lean meats and seafood make your mouth water. Essential fatty acids are yummy. (Okay, that may be going a bit too far.) Be sure to add in savory spices, seasonings, condiments, and sauces.

What's great about eating for glycemic index weight loss:

- Most gourmet food is low glycemic.

- Standard restaurant offerings include meat and seafood dishes, vegetables, and salads—exactly what you want to eat.

- Most of your friends won't even notice that you're eating differently. After all, you don't need to ask the waiter to prepare food differently or bring you special food.

- You can skip over the high-glycemic side foods like bread, sodas, and white potatoes.

- You'll eat with the joy and gratitude that glycemic index weight loss works for you

Let glycemic index weight loss rest lightly on your days. You'll feel good and look great, so enjoy.

Setting the Best Eating Mood

Realistically, you're a busy person. Your time matters to you. You eat lunch in between answering the phone and managing your e-mail or in between household chores, carpools, and running errands. Your life is busy, and your meals are mostly rushed. It's easy just to grab something convenient and quick to eat, which could be part of the reason you're on a program to lose weight. This method of eating isn't working and it is definitely fattening.

Being busy when you are eating is definitely not sensuous and pleasurable. It increases anxiety and worsens digestion. By following a glycemic index weight-loss program, however, you have a wonderful opportunity to pause and experience day-to-day eating in a different way. A more relaxing way. By now you've discovered the following things about glycemic index weight loss:

- ◆ You need to stock your kitchen with low-glycemic foods and snacks and plan your eating with them in mind. You can't just grab junk food and call it a meal.

- ◆ Eating slowly is its own reward. It takes more time to chew vegetables and meats than to inhale a burger and fries. You'll digest better, reduce stress, and enjoy your food more.

- ◆ Keep low-glycemic snack foods in your car and in your office desk. Unless you have truly enlightened office snack machine offerings, rely on your own food choices.

- ◆ The spirit of eating for glycemic index weight loss is balanced, centered, and thoughtful. Forget frantic and fearfulness. Let your body luxuriate in the wonderful food.

Your eating habits are already changing to support being at your ideal size for life. The following sections offer suggestions for making mealtimes more sensuous and pleasurable.

Lower the Stress Level

Eating when you're stressed isn't fun, and it's not great for your body. When your stress level is high, your body is in fight-or-flight mode. Your parasympathetic nervous system, which controls digestion, shuts down. When this happens, you're likely to experience indigestion or stomach discomfort. When stressed, your pleasure-sensing abilities diminish. You'll enjoy your meals much more if you decompress and de-stress before you take that first bite. Here are some suggestions for de-stressing before meals:

- ◆ Stretch or do some light movement, such as taking a walk.

- ◆ Listen to music you love and sing along.

Wrong Weigh _____

Don't let anyone disrupt your time for eating. Arguments, controversies, problems, bad moods, and discipline issues can wait until after the meal.

- Have a cup of herbal or decaffeinated tea.
- Chat with family and friends.
- Say grace with intention and thankfulness.

Create emotional and physical distance between your eating and other matters of your life. That way, when you do sit down to eat, you'll be able to focus on your food and give it your full attention.

Set the Atmosphere

Do you think of your personal eating environments as having an atmosphere? A restaurant owner knows that atmosphere can make or break a restaurant's success, regardless of how good the food is. Are you planning your eating scenario the same way a restaurant carefully plans its atmosphere?

Take a few moments to analyze your ideal eating environment and set it up for your weight-loss success. Follow these suggestions:

- Eat in a beautiful environment. Avoid eating at your desk or where you're working. Don't eat in your car. Instead, eat outside at a picnic table or at the dining room or kitchen table.

- Remove all clutter from the table and instead set the table with placemats, flatware, flowers, and candles to create a harmonious environment. Set your table with small to medium-size plates, glasses, mugs, and utensils. Avoid the large plates that invite large portions.

- Remove all clutter from your line of sight. That means dirty pots and pans, paperwork, and lists of chores to complete.

- Don't eat in front of the television. Turn it off. If you really want to watch a show that's on during dinnertime, record it to view later.

- Listen to pleasant music or engage in uplifting, interesting, or fun conversation.

- Put your food on your plate, in a pattern based on the Plate Method, before you bring it to the table. Don't put serving dishes on the table; you could be tempted to overeat.

- Before you sit down at the table, take a few moments to clear your mind from concerns and problems. Take a couple of deep breaths to release stress.

◆ Avoid discussing challenging or stressful topics while eating.

◆ If someone at the table misbehaves or is unpleasant, put down your fork and wait until the situation improves. Try not to get involved in the situation yourself.

If you're feeling stressed, it's not the time to eat, it's time to relax. Learn more about managing stress on a glycemic index weight-loss program in Chapter 23.

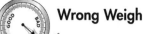

Wrong Weigh _____

If you use eating as a way to soothe stress, it's time to make a change. Find a substitute activity such as exercise, reading, walking, or a hobby. Get to the root of your stressful feelings and make the necessary personal or lifestyle changes.

Eat Slowly

Eating slowly is always a good strategy. It will even help you keep your weight off. Ideally, a meal should take a minimum of 15 to 20 minutes—but preferably longer. Most of us eat way too fast. Slowing down offers many benefits:

◆ You have to be relaxed and mindful to eat slowly and chew your food completely.

◆ You have more time in which to actually taste and enjoy your food.

◆ Your digestion improves.

◆ You can feel your stomach's hunger numbers best when you eat slowly. When you eat quickly, it's more difficult to feel stomach satisfaction.

◆ Your food lasts longer so it seems as if you're eating more food, even though you aren't.

◆ You may not have time to eat all your food, in which case, either toss it out or store it for later.

THIN-couragement _____

Learn to eat slowly by eating with a friend who eats really slowly. Eat more slowly than your friend, even if you need to match her or him bite for bite. This may drive you crazy at first, but you'll learn how to slow down at meals.

Slow eating is a reward in and of itself. You'll more than double your pleasure.

Reduce Distractions

Meals aren't pleasurable when you have lots of distractions. Not only are distractions annoying, they make it difficult to focus on enjoying your food. Here are some suggestions to eliminate distractions:

◆ Turn off the phone or don't answer it.

◆ Turn off the media—computers, cell phones, television, computer games, and radio (unless you are listening to background music).

◆ Don't answer the doorbell unless you expect company.

◆ Don't engage in arguments or controversies with your children or other family members.

THIN-couragement

When you eat at a fine restaurant, you expect good service and no distractions. In fact, part of the price includes eating in a serene and beautiful environment. As best you can, create the same relaxing and calm ambience when you eat at home.

Depending on your family and their needs, reducing all distractions is impossible. For example, babies can be fussy, and teenagers can be late to dinner. But within the realm of practicality, make your meals pleasant.

Eat Sitting Down

Stand-up eating was once considered impolite. But that was many years ago, before our national population was 67 percent overweight and expanding daily. Sitting down when you eat doesn't guarantee you'll be healthier and it won't make you automatically thinner, but it sure helps.

Wrong Weigh

Before you put that first bite of food into your mouth, sit down. Do this for every taste while you're cooking and for every morsel of food you want to eat when you're clearing the dishes. Sit to eat and you'll find that you won't be eating as much food as before.

Sitting down helps you relax and makes you aware that you're eating. Stand-up eating is often mindless, as when a person is snacking while cooking dinner or when standing in front of the sink looking out the kitchen window.

Be sure you don't eat standing up at a party, at the ball game, or at a backyard barbeque. Usually, when people eat while standing up, they eat faster and the foods they eat tend to be fast food or junk food. Seldom do people eat grilled salmon and salad when standing up. But they do eat chips, sodas, appetizers, crackers, candy, and all the high-carb snack foods.

Three Meals a Day and More

One eating custom is virtually universal, practiced in nearly every culture around the world: eating three meals a day—breakfast, lunch, and dinner. This commonality suggests that we all experience stomach hunger at least three times a day.

On the glycemic index weight-loss program, be sure to eat at least three times a day, especially breakfast. Avoid skipping meals, because that can make your blood sugar levels and insulin levels unstable. Skipping meals also slows your metabolism—the very thing you don't want to happen.

Perhaps you've heard that snacking is bad for you. Not true. If you're hungry between meals, you can have a snack. Just make sure you include your snack in your total glycemic load intake for the day.

THIN-couragement

When Molly wanted a snack, she made sure she ate low-glycemic foods, but she wasn't gaining any sustenance from the snack. Instead she was gaining weight. Her typical snack consisted of a caffeinated diet soda and three or four artificially sweetened gelatin desserts. There wasn't any food in her snack. The caffeine triggered a rise in blood sugar levels, resulting in a rise in insulin levels. Eating that much artificial sweetener was also inhibiting her weight loss, and causing her to gain weight.

Eat snacks that are nutritionally balanced. For example, half an avocado with salad dressing, a handful of nuts and an ounce of hard cheese, a hard-boiled egg with a teaspoon of real mayonnaise, or a turkey and cheese roll-up. Eat regular food for snacks that are low in carbohydrates and high in nutrition.

Late-Night Eating

Late-night eating is in a whole different category than snacking. Raiding the refrigerator at night is fattening and often a sign of unfulfilled emotional needs. Most late-night eating is ...

- **Mindless.** It's unplanned and not factored into a person's daily glycemic index eating program.

◆ **Emotional eating.** We've never heard of anyone who favors taking broiled fish filets to bed for a midnight snack. Instead, they choose high-starch, high-sugar, and high-carbohydrate comfort foods.

Avoid late-night eating. If you want a snack before bed, that's fine, but after you get into bed, don't eat until morning unless you have a doctor's written permission to do so.

The Least You Need to Know

◆ Use simple stress-reduction techniques to decompress before you start eating.

◆ Create an eating environment that's appealing, calm, and relaxing.

◆ Eat three meals a day plus snacks.

◆ Eat slowly and sit while eating.

◆ Enjoy eating the delicious foods as part of your glycemic index weight-loss program.

Chapter **18**

Eating Out

In This Chapter

- ◆ Ordering at a restaurant
- ◆ Eating low glycemic at fast-food restaurants
- ◆ Dining at friends' homes
- ◆ Understanding restaurant menus
- ◆ Analyzing restaurant appetizers, entrées, and desserts

Dining out on a glycemic index weight-loss program is easier than you probably think. The rumors that it's hard were once true, but no longer. You know what to eat on a glycemic index weight-loss program, and now some of the people who plan restaurant menus are also clued in.

They want you to eat out and they want you to eat out often. Sure, you may need to eat less of some special whole-grain breads and other unique foods, but eating out, dining out, going through the drive-through, or eating at the buffet has never been easier.

This chapter guides you through the process of ordering meals at restaurants. You learn how and what to order and how to negotiate with the waitperson. You also learn how to eat at friends' homes and stay true to your glycemic index way of eating.

Restaurants

The fundamental ingredients of glycemic index eating are the basic foods that make up most restaurant meals. Meats, fish, poultry, vegetables, and fruit are all-time standards. Provided that a restaurant offers those basics, it can serve you food to meet your weight-loss needs.

If you view glycemic index eating this way, you can be comfortable ordering a meal in virtually any restaurant. You don't need to be intimidated—remember, the restaurant is there to meet your needs, not the other way around.

Wrong Weigh _____

Finding balanced, low-glycemic meals can be challenging at two types of restaurants. The first is at vegetarian restaurants, especially if they don't serve any animal proteins, such as meat or fish. The second is, surprisingly, salad bars. Often, salad bars skimp on their offerings of animal protein and instead offer bits of meat or fish in pasta salads and serve up shredded hard cheeses. If you can find a salad bar where you can eat three ounces of high-quality animal protein at a meal, or hard-boiled eggs, then go ahead and eat there. If not, pass on these types of restaurants.

Ordering from the Menu

Let's make ordering as easy as possible. For all meals—breakfasts, lunches and dinners—start with an entrée. Bypass the pastas and pizzas, and let your eyes cruise through the salads, entrées, and sandwiches.

Yes, we said sandwiches. Sandwiches can offer delicious combinations of meats and cheeses. However, it's highly unlikely that a sandwich shop will have low-glycemic bread. When you order a sandwich, ask the server to hold the bread. They know how to do this. Also ask whether you can substitute a small salad or fruit for french fries or chips.

If you love bread, eat at restaurants and delis that offer stone-ground whole-wheat or sourdough bread, and have your sandwich made with one of those.

Think of menus as guidelines and not as cast in concrete. Ask for low-glycemic side dishes such as salads or fruit, dressing on the side, no dressing, or oil and vinegar. You can also request special preparation techniques if you want to eat low-fat meals. The waiter's job is to serve you. If he or she doesn't, choose a different restaurant next time.

Select the main-dish salad or entrée that sounds the best. If you want an appetizer, order one that contains vegetables and meats and skip the ones with high amounts of starches or fat, such as quesadillas, corn-bread, or fried cheese.

Tossed salads and main-dish salads always work for glycemic index weight loss, as do sautéed or steamed vegetables. If you want the artichoke cheese dip as an appetizer, be sure to ask the server to bring cut vegetables instead of crackers or bread for dipping.

Desserts can be a nice finish to a meal. Order dessert provided that you …

- ◆ Have room left in your stomach. Don't forget the 0–5 rule.

- ◆ Have room left in your glycemic load for the day.

- ◆ Have confidence that you can stop at just a couple bites and ask the waiter to take away the rest.

- ◆ Can share the dessert with others at the table.

Wrong Weigh

Most french fries are still fried in oils that contain trans fats. Until the perfect cooking oil is created, french fries have two strikes against them: they're high glycemic and the trans fats are especially bad for your heart. Take a pass.

THIN-couragement

You don't need to explain to the server that you are eating based on the glycemic index unless you want to. Sometimes it might seem helpful, but as you gather experience and confidence, ordering will become second nature to you.

A taste is as satisfying to your taste buds as a portion. And you'll definitely like the long-term results more.

Don't Super-Size

Super-sized meals are way too big for you. They're too big for anyone. They contain too much food of questionable value. Don't order them. Instead, half-size your meals by sharing your entrée with a friend or ordering the junior burger.

Most restaurant portions are huge—big enough for two and sometimes even large enough for three people. That is, unless you are eating at a very fine—meaning expensive—restaurant. Only then do the portion sizes relate in any way to the size of your stomach—the same size as your fist.

You can stretch your "eat-out" budget while eating a right-size meal. Share the entrée and meal with a friend. Restaurant servers are great at handling this situation. Often, they split the entrées and side salads in the kitchen, sometimes adding a nominal split-plate charge.

THIN-couragement

> Suzi and Jack always share an entrée when they eat out at restaurants, and even sometimes at fast-food places. They each get plenty to eat and often they end up taking some food home—usually enough for one person's lunch the next day. They spend less and actually enjoy leaving the table feeling comfortable and not stuffed.

At the Buffet

You may find it trickier to navigate your way through a buffet line than at a "sit-down and be served" restaurant. Too many choices, too much food, and often, but not always, way too many high-glycemic choices.

There are exceptions. Some Sunday buffet brunches are simply wonderful. They offer vegetables, salads, eggs, and meats. When they are truly elaborate, you can eat seafood, Eggs Benedict (hold the muffin unless it's sourdough or stone-ground whole wheat), and delightful fruit. Your challenge is to only put the foods on your plate that look most appealing and to be highly discerning about the foods you don't want to eat.

But most family buffet restaurants are more challenging. Here's how to approach the buffet line. Go backward. Survey the line starting at the end, where the good stuff is, such as prime rib and salmon. Then walk toward the front of the line, planning which foods to put on your plate. Remember, your tummy has a limited amount of room. Following are tips for getting through the line:

◆ On your first pass, avoid filling up your plate with foods placed at the start of the line. They're usually the inexpensive and least nutritious filler foods. Instead, save room on your plate for the best foods placed toward the end of the line. Take the plate back to your seat and eat slowly and sensuously. Remember, at the buffet there is always plenty of food.

◆ If and only if you have more room in your stomach, take a second walk through the line, taking morsels and bites or even seconds of some of your favorites.

◆ Ignore high-glycemic—white or fluffy—pastries, cereals, and breads. Train yourself not to see them until you develop a true understanding of how they affect your body. They're what other people may choose to eat, not what you eat.

◆ If there's any room left in your stomach, ask for a bite of a friend's dessert. Or just order tea or coffee and finish your meal with a light feeling in your stomach.

Use this same technique for buffets at holiday parties and summer picnics. Just because it's on the table doesn't mean it needs to be in your mouth or stomach. Now that many people are also eating based on the glycemic index, you may find yourself delighted with the offerings at potluck dinners and tailgate parties.

Fast Food

They're everywhere—on virtually every city street corner and at stops along the highway. They're convenient. They offer inexpensive food. So what's the problem?

The most popular menu offerings at fast-food restaurants are high glycemic, high in fat, and high in high-fructose corn syrup or artificial sweeteners. They offer all the eating components you want to avoid. But—and here's the good news—things are changing in the fast-food world, and they're changing fast.

Fast-food restaurants want to meet your needs—they want your business—so they now offer menu choices based on the glycemic index. Here are some suggestions for eating fast food that's low in carbohydrates:

◆ Order a hamburger or cheeseburger (hold the bun) with a small salad. Ask for a glass of water. This meal is farm sourced.

◆ Never "super-size" anything.

◆ If everyone else wants pizza, go ahead and order it with a salad. Eat the salad. You can also have a slice or two of pizza, but eat your pizza differently. Peel off the topping and eat it. Toss out the crust. You are able to eat the best part of the pizza and savor the taste.

◆ Order a submarine sandwich in either a wrap or bread. Also ask for a fork and knife. Have your sandwich prepared with all the salad toppings. Open up the sandwich or wrap and eat the insides with fork and knife. If the shop will "hold" the bread, ask them to do that.

◆ Order the main-dish salad. Use some of the salad dressing. You might want to pass on the croutons and crunchy noodles. The salad by itself is low glycemic, but the added condiments could be high glycemic.

- We haven't seen any beverage offerings that are completely suitable for a glycemic index weight-loss program. They are full of high-fructose corn syrup, aspartame, sucralose, or caffeine. Even an 8-ounce glass of juice could have too high a glycemic value for you. Your best beverage choice as of this writing is plain water or herbal tea.

- Enjoy fried chicken by removing the skin before you eat it. Before you eat the coleslaw, drain off some of the sugary liquid. Pass on the biscuits and mashed potatoes. Absolutely pass on the honey blend; it contains less honey and more high-fructose corn syrup.

- Eat the fillings of tacos and burritos with a fork and pass on the tortillas. Ditto with taco salads.

As you eat at fast-food restaurants, you're going to find more menu choices based on the glycemic index. Be sure to read the fine print before you indulge. Remember, you can't go wrong with a burger (hold the bun) and a salad.

At a Friend's Home

Eating based on the glycemic index at a friend's home could be tricky. Perhaps you've had people over for dinner and noticed that one person wasn't eating. You find out too late that the person is allergic to the foods you offered or was for some other reason unable to eat them. Gosh, how you wish that person had phoned you ahead of time and discussed his or her dietary needs. It would have saved both of you embarrassing discomfort.

Here are some suggestions for eating based on the glycemic index at a friend's home:

- Call ahead and ask whether you can bring a dish or beverage. That way, you can bring foods or beverages that fit into your glycemic index eating program.

- Call ahead at least a week in advance and tell your host or hostess of any food allergies you have. Include special food needs.

- If your host or hostess asks whether you have any food preferences, keep your answer simple. Basically, you can eat meat, fish, and vegetables. So say that and avoid elaborate requests. You want to be invited back, and getting food-fussy at a party isn't fun for anyone.

◆ If worse comes to worst, you can pick at your food, claim not to be hungry, and then eat later on the way home.

◆ Most hosts offer some form of meat, seafood, or poultry and some vegetables, so eat what you can.

Eating meals at a friend's home isn't really about the food, it's about the friendship and good times. Don't let the food get in the way. Eat ahead, eat at the party, eat after the party, but make the most of your friendships. They'll last long after you've attained your ideal size.

Take-Along Food

Now that you're eating very differently, don't get caught without food when you need it. Perhaps you decided to head out shopping at about 3 P.M. After an hour, you're starving. You need food and you need it now. What are you going to do?

It's really easy to find unacceptable foods at malls and shopping areas. But you don't want to eat candy, cinnamon rolls, doughy hot pretzels, sugary beverages, or cookies. Let's face it—food vendors at the malls don't sell hard-boiled eggs, carrot sticks, or raw fruit.

This is the time when you need to be your own best friend. Never leave home without some kinds of acceptable foods. Keep these foods in your glove compartment, handbag, backpack, or briefcase. You can also keep them in your desk at work. Acceptable snacks include the following:

◆ Small containers of hard cheese that don't require refrigeration.

◆ Small containers of peanut butter that don't require refrigeration.

◆ Nuts, such as pecans, peanuts, hazelnuts, cashews, and almonds.

◆ Dried apricots are low glycemic, as are dried pears, peaches, and apples.

THIN**-couragement**

Wouldn't it be great to be able to order a cup of herbal tea at a fast-food restaurant? Until that day, take a tea bag with you and order a cup of hot water.

THIN**-couragement**

Use an insulated container to carry foods for more culinary variety. That way you can carry salads with cottage cheese, poultry, and meat.

- Small cans of tuna or sardines. Pack along a plastic fork and paper napkin.

- Beef or buffalo jerky, homemade or made without preservatives and artificial coloring.

- Raw carrots, celery, radishes, and other raw vegetables.

Body of Knowledge

You may have read or heard that carrots are high glycemic, but they aren't. Early testing methods found them to be high, but it simply wasn't reasonable that the only high-glycemic vegetable was carrots. Recent tests show them to be low, whether cooked or raw.

- Water. If you are in your car frequently, tote along a stainless-steel water bottle filled with purified water. Often a glass of water can ease hunger for a half hour until you can find a place to eat. Using a stainless-steel water bottle (purchase at the health-food store, sporting goods store, or www.amazon.com) lets you avoid the plastic bottle health, environmental, and recycling concerns.

- Black or green olives in a waterproof container.

- Coarsely ground low-glycemic whole-grain products such as crackers and bread. You can also add some al dente whole-grain pasta to your salads.

As you eat snacks, remember to only eat when your stomach is hungry—at a 0—and to stop eating at or below a 5—at comfortable. By packing these kinds of food items and eating them when you get hungry, you can avoid becoming so hungry that you want to eat a horse—that is, a horse made of sugar and dough.

The Least You Need to Know

- You can always eat low glycemic by ordering animal proteins and vegetables— hold the breads and desserts.

- Don't be intimidated by restaurant servers—their job is to serve you the foods that you want to eat.

- Fast-food restaurants now offer main-dish salads and side salads that work for the glycemic index weight-loss program.

- Carry low-glycemic snacks with you so that you never need to resort to eating unacceptable foods when hungry.

Shopping Based on the Glycemic Index

In This Chapter

◆ Selecting grocery store foods

◆ Buying meats and vegetables

◆ Selecting packaged foods

◆ Frequenting your health-food store

You've spent years knowing exactly how to shop for groceries. You may have even memorized what to purchase from each aisle, and you certainly know how to shop the specials. So who would have thought you would ever need to relearn such a basic skill as grocery shopping?

As you read this book, your shopping habits are changing. You're reading product ingredient lists and you know how many processed and high-glycemic carbohydrates are found in seemingly innocent foods. Little did you realize just how many high-glycemic foods you once ate on a daily basis.

In this chapter, you learn guidelines for how to shop for glycemic index weight loss and for weight maintenance. You'll find the new way of shopping just as easy as before, and you'll find new foods and be able to experience new culinary delights.

At the Grocery Store

As you review your weekly glycemic index weight-loss grocery-shopping list, here's what you're going to find. Most of the foods on your list are available at the outside perimeter of the store, in the frozen-food section, or in the health-food section. In fact, with the exception of condiments, spices, herbal teas, olive oil, vinegar, and household items, you never need to walk down the food aisles packed full with carbohydrate-rich foods.

It's possible that you won't find some of the items on your list at the grocery store at all, in which case you'll need to visit a health-food store once or twice a month. How to shop at health-food stores is discussed later in this chapter. The following sections discuss how to shop at the grocery store.

> **Body of Knowledge**
>
> The fat in beef is less saturated today than it was 10 years ago. Many cattle are now both range-fed and grain-fed, which results in less saturated fat in the meat. Ten years ago, most cattle were only grain-fed.

> **THIN-couragement**
>
> Always keep a few pounds of lean ground beef in your freezer. With a pound of ground beef you can make hamburgers, tacos for Mexican main courses, or Italian meat sauce to serve with spaghetti squash or a half cup of whole-wheat al dente pasta. You can even serve it over cooked cauliflower—believe it or not, it tastes great.

Shopping for Animal Protein

You have many choices for animal protein that give you great taste and can also be easy on your budget. Animal protein is zero on the glycemic index.

Beef. This food is a reliable pleaser and is highly versatile for your glycemic index weight-loss program. Your choices include cuts that cook up quickly on the grill, such as lean ground beef and steaks, roasts for the oven or slow-cooker, precut strips for sautéing, and flank steak to marinate and cook on the grill or in the oven.

Don't forget sliced all-natural roast beef, ham, or turkey from the deli counter to eat for breakfast or lunchtime roll-ups and as late-afternoon snacks. You can even serve them warmed up with eggs for breakfast. You can also roast beef, ham, or turkey at home and slice for sandwiches and snacks.

Pork. Pork adds variety and many pork cuts are low in fat, such as pork chops, tenderloin, ham, and roasts. Pork ribs are excellent—slow-cook to render off the fat, and then crisp up in the oven or on the grill. Pork sausage tends to be very fatty, so you may want to pass on it and select turkey sausage instead. But be sure to check the labels, because some turkey sausage is also quite high in fat. By trimming off excess fat, you can more easily keep your daily fat intake at 30 percent of your food.

> **Wrong Weigh**
>
> If you are purchasing your meats at the butcher's counter, be sure to ask the butcher to trim all visible fat from the meat before he or she wraps it. This saves you time and spares you the temptation of eating more fat than you need.

Chicken and turkey. Poultry readily picks up the flavors of other foods, such as condiments, spices, and any vegetables it's cooked with. Grocery stores offer a wide variety of prepackaged choices: drumsticks, breasts, strips for fajitas, and breast pieces for stews and quick sautéing. Purchase whole turkeys or just the turkey breast for roasting. You'll have meat left over for cold cuts and snacks.

Specialty meats. Don't forget to consider cooking with lamb, veal, and Cornish game hens. Many people favor buffalo and game, such as duck, pheasant, and elk. You can find many excellent low-glycemic recipes for specialty meats.

Seafood. Shellfish and fish taste best when purchased fresh and eaten within a day. You can also freeze them, if you need to. Avoid purchasing seafood that's already been frozen and then thawed. You need to eat it right away, and you can't refreeze it. If you can't find fresh-caught fish, purchase it frozen and store it in your freezer until you're ready to thaw and cook it.

Eggs. Plan to always keep eggs on hand. Sauté some for breakfast or hard-boil them for brown-bag lunches and tuna or salmon salads. Eggs stay fresh for weeks in your refrigerator.

Canned and prepackaged fish and meats. Think tuna, salmon, and sardines. These are available in cans and prepackaged in plastic and foil bags. Keep some on hand for traveling, snacks, and quick lunches or breakfasts. Canned salmon and tuna are usually caught wild.

Bacon. A few slices a couple of times a month is a treat. Bacon only contains about two grams of protein per slice, so you need to add other protein to your meal to eat the recommended 15 to 20 grams of animal protein per meal. Purchase the kind of bacon you like best. Because bacon is very high in saturated fat, use it sparingly. Be sure to pour off the fat before you serve it and toss out the rendered fat. You can also purchase turkey bacon. It tastes great, too. Be sure to read the fat content on the label to make sure the turkey bacon is indeed lower in fat. Sometimes it's not.

THIN -couragement

> For an occasional tasty treat, you can purchase thinly sliced salami. To cook, spread on paper towels on a microwavable plate. Microwave on high for 15 seconds or until the salami is crisp. It's great for snacks and also good crumbled up in salads. One slice or two per family-size salad is plenty for flavor and is very satisfying. And, good news, most of the fat is absorbed by the paper towels.

At the Deli

Consider the deli to be your quick-meal resource center. You can purchase whole roasted chickens and a wide variety of sliced meats and cheeses. You may want to pass on the salads because they tend to be high in processed starches and sugars. Definitely avoid salads made with white pastas, grains, and flavored gelatin. Instead, look for tossed vegetable salads and coleslaws. Whole roasted chicken is often available and a good choice.

Vegetables

So many vegetables, such little time. If you're like most people in the vegetable section of the grocery store, you buy the same vegetables over and over again and never even think to try something new. Now is the time to shop this section with new eyes.

You'll find snow peapods, fennel root, celery root, and spaghetti squash. And that's just a start. Now that you are eating 5 to 10 servings of vegetables and fruits a day, widen your choices. Cooking directions are usually on the labels, and if not, ask the produce experts at the store. Here are some tips about purchasing vegetables:

- ◆ Purchase fresh or frozen. Fresh vegetables keep about a week in the vegetable crisper of your refrigerator. Frozen keep much longer. Keep frozen vegetables as a backup in case you run out of fresh produce during the week.

- Frozen vegetables are a great choice because they are frozen at optimal ripeness. Fresh produce is often harvested weeks before it arrives at the grocer's shelves and may have lost important nutrients in transit.

- Prepackaged lettuces and vegetables that are cleaned and cut are convenient, but perhaps cost more. The baby carrots and trimmed romaine hearts may be worth it. If you want convenience, shop the prepackaged sections.

- Use spices and condiments to jazz up vegetables. Try a sprinkle of dried tarragon on cauliflower, curry on broccoli, and cilantro on tomatoes. The spices and herbs bring out the flavor of vegetables. Eat them plain or eat them spiced, but be sure to eat them.

- Purchase or grow fresh herbs to add to salads. Chopped fresh basil, tarragon, parsley, cilantro, and others add zest and interest to a tossed green salad. You can find sun-dried tomatoes in the produce section. Add a mere teaspoon in sauces, meat, or over vegetables to give them a delicious Mediterranean flavor.

Vegetables give your mouth and stomach satisfaction. Eaten raw, they're crunchy and have plenty of fiber. Cook your vegetables to the al dente stage, meaning still a bit crunchy, so that you enjoy the mouth satisfaction that vegetables offer.

In the summer and fall, you can purchase vegetables and fruit at local farmers' markets that are held in most communities. Usually, the produce is locally grown and picked fresh. Take cash, because you may not be able to pay with a credit card. Going to a farmers' market allows you to support local growers and get fresh produce weekly.

Fruit

Fruit is nature's candy. It tastes sweet, satisfies your sweet tooth, and is full of important nutrients and antioxidants. Plus, fruit is mostly low glycemic with some being medium glycemic.

Choose more common fruits, such as apples, oranges, and pears, or shop for more exotic fare, such as pomegranates and papayas. When eating, savor the natural sweetness, texture, and juiciness of the fruit. Purchase organic when you can.

$\mathcal{THIN}$ **-couragement** _____

In many parts of the country, it's hard to purchase fresh berries that are ripe and mold-free. If you live in one of those areas, use frozen berries. Find them unsweetened in resealable plastic bags in the freezer section of the grocery store. They're yummy and delicious eaten plain or in a glass parfait with whipped low-fat cream cheese. Or place frozen in a blender to make a thick frosty dessert. Plus, berries are low glycemic.

Cheese

Grocery stores now offer a wide and delicious selection of world-class and exotic cheeses from around the country and the planet. Ditto with health-food stores and natural-food grocers. At some, you can sample and discuss your selections with a cheese specialist.

Choose your favorite hard or soft cheeses, such as cheddar, Brie, cream cheese, and Parmesan. In a sense, the world's the limit on what cheeses you can enjoy. Cheese is low glycemic.

$\mathcal{THIN}$ **-couragement** _____

Shredded and shaved Parmesan cheese is almost mandatory as a kitchen staple, right up there with salt, pepper, and olive oil. Add a bit of shaved Parmesan to eggs, salads, and cooked vegetables. Add shredded Parmesan to cottage cheese and sprinkle over spaghetti sauce. It's salty and tangy, so just a little bit will go far in expanding the aroma and enhancing the flavor of your meal.

Whole Grains and Cereals

Get ready to read the list of ingredients. Here's what to look for:

◆ **Brown rice.** This rice is already a whole grain and it has more fiber and more nutrients than white rice. Wild rice is a good choice and is a grass, not a grain, but you cook and serve it just as you would regular rice. When you purchase rice, check out the glycemic index of that variety of rice. The glycemic indexes of rice range from low to high. Basmati is low, sticky white rice is high.

◆ **Whole-grain pasta.** The whole-grain variety is now available in most grocery stores. Remember to cook it to barely al dente for low-glycemic eating.

◆ **Corn tortillas and whole-wheat tortillas.** Corn tortillas are medium glycemic, and some whole-wheat and white wheat tortillas are high glycemic.

◆ **Breads.** If you can find true coarsely ground whole-grain bread, buy it. But most store-bought breads contain finely milled enriched or white flour, as well as sugars and some mystery ingredients. If the bread, muffin, hard roll, or hamburger bun isn't made with 100 percent whole-wheat flour, pass on it. If it's finely milled, pass on it. Some specialty bread shops and grocery stores now offer truly whole-grain breads. Stone-ground bread is your best choice and tastes best, too. It's flavorful and slightly earthy. While most whole-wheat and white-wheat breads are high glycemic, authentic stone-ground breads are medium.

Wrong Weigh

Caramel coloring is often added to breads and bread products to make them appear healthier; that is, to contain more whole wheat than they do. Don't buy bread with caramel coloring. Instead look for bread that is truly 100 percent stone-ground grain.

◆ **Cookies, cakes, and other baked goods.** It's unlikely that any of these products are totally whole grain. Most cookies and cakes are medium-glycemic because they're made with butter or oil, which lowers the glycemic index value. Consider them to be factory sourced and eat sparingly provided that your glycemic load stays in range for the meal and the day.

◆ **Cereals.** With the exception of All-Bran, muesli, some Kashi cereals, and steel-cut oats, breakfast cereals are high or medium glycemic and are often filled with refined or enriched flours and grains. The fluffier the cereal, the higher glycemic. Added sugar makes it even higher glycemic. Breakfast cereals are factory sourced, so read labels to assure that you're purchasing the purest. Due to the high glycemic factor of many breakfast cereals, you may want to eat eggs or meat with vegetables and fruit for breakfast and pass on factory-sourced breakfast cereals.

◆ **Other grains.** Barley, wheat berries, rye kernels, cracked wheat, and buckwheat groats are grains you may enjoy. If you can't find them at the grocery store, you can purchase them at health-food stores. These grains are low-glycemic products.

When selecting and eating grains and cereals, be sure you don't overeat them. Eat them sparingly, still focusing on making protein and vegetables the mainstay of your meals and snacks.

Dairy, Nuts, and Other Foods

Many grocers now offer large packages of nuts in the produce section: pecans, pistachios, Brazil nuts, hazelnuts, cashews, almonds, walnuts, pinions, peanuts, and more. Overall, they're a better buy than the small packages of nuts in the baking section. Use nuts for snacks and salad toppings. Process them into nut flour in the food processor to replace flour in cookie and cake recipes. Process them beyond the flour phase to create nut butters. Almonds, peanuts, hazelnuts, and cashews are delicious.

Pickles, capers, vinegars, anchovies, horseradish, and other condiments make good recipes even better. As these are generally low glycemic (one exception is sweet pickles), have fun with your shopping and eating.

THIN -couragement

Stock up on acidic condiments, such as dill pickles, capers, mustards, chutney, onions, vinegars, sauerkraut, horseradish, and marinated vegetables such as mushrooms and artichoke hearts. Choose tangy salsas made without sugars and select bottles of authentic lemon or lime juice. Eat these with your meals to naturally lower the glycemic load of the meal.

Oils and Butter

Use olive oil for dressing salads and light sautéing, and cooking. It's really the only oil you need in your pantry. If you want more variety, purchase only *cold-expeller pressed* vegetable or nut oils, such as walnut oil or canola oil. You'll find a wider selection at health-food stores and fancier grocery stores.

Glyco Lingo

Cold-expeller pressed oils are extracted from vegetables or nuts without using heat, but only through pressing. When heat is used to extract oils, the heat can damage the essential fatty acids contained in the oil.

Use butter to melt on vegetables, for sautéing, and for cooking at higher heats. Nothing tastes better in baked goods than butter. Butter is farm sourced. Don't purchase margarines and fake butters. They aren't as versatile and could contain mystery ingredients and partially hydrogenated vegetable oils because they're factory sourced. If you have concerns about your heart health and have been advised by a health practitioner to cut back on butter, substitute with olive oil if you can.

At the Health-Food Store

If you haven't already visited, it's time to become familiar with your local health-food store. Not just the part of the store that's filled with vitamins and supplements, but the natural-foods section that offers baked goods, cheeses, bulk nuts, meats, eggs, and legumes.

Put these foods on your health-food store shopping list:

◆ Bulk psyllium to increase your fiber intake and for proper elimination. Psyllium is a zero-glycemic grain with no calories. To use, add 1 tablespoon psyllium to a large glass of water and drink immediately. Follow up with another glass of water.

◆ Bulk flax seeds. To obtain the highest nutritional benefit, grind the flax seeds just before eating but you can also receive nutritional value from eating them whole. Flax seeds can be ground in a small coffee grinder at home. After grinding, store in the freezer to protect the valuable omega-3 fatty acids from becoming rancid. Sprinkle on salads, eggs, and vegetables. Don't use for cooking or baking as heat can damage the valuable essential fatty acid content.

◆ Whole grains. These often come in bulk bins. Use for pilafs and side dishes.

◆ Steel-cut oats (also called thick-cut or Irish oats on some packages). Make hot cereal with these oats. The cooking time is about 20 to 30 minutes.

◆ Wild rice. It often costs less at health-food stores. Wild rice adds sparkle and a depth of taste when added to rice before cooking.

◆ Dried fruit in bulk, like apricots, pears, peaches, raisins, dates, cherries, cranberries, strawberries, blueberries, figs, pineapple, papaya, and others. Many packaged dried fruits contain sulfur dioxide, which can cause sensitivity in some individuals. Bulk dried fruits tend not to contain sulfur dioxide or other additives. Add dried fruit to nuts and seeds for trail mix, sprinkle in tossed salads, or add to pilafs, dressings, and sauces.

◆ Organic milk, yogurt, and butter. Comes from the milk of dairy cows that aren't raised with hormones and steroids.

◆ Specialty cheeses.

◆ Nuts and spices in bulk.

Health-food stores may have higher prices than grocery stores, so shop selectively. Read the grocery store and health-food store promotional fliers every week so you can take advantage of meat and fish specials, as well as specials on frozen vegetables and fruit. You can also find grocery coupons at www.coupons.com and others.

The Least You Need to Know

◆ Glycemic index weight loss lets you develop new grocery-shopping habits.

◆ Purchase most foods around the perimeter of the grocery store and only some in the aisles.

◆ Select either fresh or frozen vegetables and fruits.

◆ Select farm-sourced foods when you can, and be cautious when purchasing factory-sourced foods.

20

Cooking Based on the Glycemic Index

In This Chapter

◆ Starting with proteins and vegetables

◆ Using recipes and cookbooks

◆ Cooking for yourself or a family

◆ Modifying recipes

◆ Packing meals and snacks

Now that you're cooking based on the glycemic index, you need a new answer to the question "What's for dinner?" Your answer might have once been, "Meat and potatoes." Or perhaps it was, "Takeout."

Your new answer is quite simple. "It will be healthy and wonderful!" The answer holds true whether you're eating takeout, cooking in, or planning a dinner party or outdoor barbeque.

Cooking based on the glycemic index might be new to you, but it's more balanced and healthy, and it's actually easier than many other ways of cooking. You'll be using protein (red meat, seafood, eggs, cheese, or poultry), small amounts of healthy fats, and lower-glycemic, mostly farm-sourced carbohydrates including vegetables, fruit, some whole grains, nuts and seeds, some dairy, and spices and condiments. When these ingredients are well prepared and thoughtfully combined, you'll have the makings of a delicious and nutritious meal.

THIN -couragement

> You can find glycemic-index cooking classes at kitchen stores and diabetic teaching centers. Call and ask for a schedule and attend some classes. You'll gather plenty of ideas you can use, plus you'll enjoy the eating.

Gustatory Delights

Somehow the very thought of meat and vegetables sounds dry and stiff, which certainly isn't appetizing. But don't let the sound fool you. The world's gourmet cuisines are low glycemic: Italian, Mexican, French, Greek, American, and Asian. Glycemic index weight-loss meals can be stunning and either simple or complex to prepare—based on your preference.

We've served glycemic index weight-loss meals to guests who have battled over licking the last drops of sauce from the bowl of a simple dish called Fennel and Tomatoes. Dinner guests have eaten every last bite of Paprika Chicken, as well as Pork Chops with Raisins and Walnuts. Try the Basil Pot Roast—you'll love it. You can find these and other recipes based on the glycemic index in *The Complete Idiot's Guide to Low-Carb Meals, The Complete Idiot's Guide to Terrific Diabetic Meals, and The Complete Idiot's Guide Glycemic Index Cookbook.*

It's easy for anyone to give up on a weight-loss program when the food is unfamiliar, odd, or extreme. Cooking for glycemic index weight loss is none of these things after you figure it out. In essence, all you're doing is substituting low-glycemic farm-sourced foods (whole, unprocessed starches and sugars) for high-glycemic or factory-sourced foods (those that are high in refined starches and sugars).

Planning Meals

Whether you like to carefully preplan your weekly meals or prepare foods more spontaneously, the following glycemic index cooking basics will work well for you:

◆ About one fourth of each meal should be from an animal protein. Think eggs, meat, seafood, poultry, or cheese for breakfast, lunch, and dinner.

◆ Add in vegetables for all meals. Prepare two or three vegetable servings per meal. Make sure that vegetables comprise about half your meal.

◆ The final fourth of the meal should consist of yams, legumes, fruit, dairy, whole-grain pasta, or rice.

◆ Use spaghetti squash to substitute for spaghetti, zucchini slices to substitute for lasagna noodles, and mashed, cooked cauliflower in place of mashed potatoes.

◆ Use lettuce leaves to hold sandwich fillings, or use cabbage or slices of jicama instead of stone ground breads if you want to keep your glycemic load low.

THIN-couragement

If you're looking for a soothing hobby, consider gardening. That way, you can grow fresh vegetables and fruit such as lettuce, strawberries, carrots, and more. You can reap the culinary rewards of your efforts, plus enjoy a creative and relaxing hobby.

◆ If you want dessert, bake or cook some recipes from the many excellent low-glycemic and low-carb cookbooks available. Be sure to avoid cooking with artificial sweeteners, because they can actually increase your appetite and promote weight gain, plus they could be harmful to your health.

◆ Get creative. Spread nut butters on slices of apples, peaches, or pears for an out-of-this-world delicious treat. Ditto on cheese.

◆ Always cook more meat for dinner than you and your family can eat. The leftovers are great for breakfast, lunch, the next night's dinner, and snacks. However, unless it's salmon or tuna, leftover fish is usually awful. You can make tuna or salmon salad with the leftovers.

Body of Knowledge

Limit low-glycemic starches to only one fourth of the space on your plate! For example, a couple of croutons on a salad and half of a small yam is about one fourth of the space on your plate. A few corn tortilla chips with guacamole salad is fine, but pass on the sopapillas (Mexican fried dessert bread made with white flour). Prepare your own croutons with sourdough bread cubes to lower the glycemic index of regular croutons.

◆ Keep cut-up carrots and celery in the refrigerator. Eat them by themselves or add some nut butter or cheese for an instant snack. You can also keep slices of radishes, jicama, green and red peppers, broccoli, cauliflower, and so on (the list is almost endless) in the refrigerator.

◆ Clean lettuce once a week, when you are putting the groceries away, to avoid needing to clean lettuce every time you prepare a salad. Use a salad spinner to remove excess water. Lettuce will keep for a week in the crisper.

◆ If you don't already have one, purchase a slow cooker. Let meats such as pork ribs, chuck roast, and pork loin simmer during the day. At dinnertime, the meat's ready to eat and all you need to do is cook some vegetables or make a tossed salad for dinner. Add a sauce to the meat, if you prefer.

◆ Use the outdoor grill as a quick way to cook meats, fish, and vegetables without needing to clean pots and pans after dinner.

◆ Keep condiments such as shredded and shaved Parmesan cheese, spices and herbs, olive oil, vinegar, sun-dried tomatoes, and garlic on hand. Also stock up on green and black olives, and cans of mushrooms and artichokes.

◆ Because acidic foods lower the glycemic index, keep plenty of acidic condiments in your pantry and refrigerator and serve them with your meals.

◆ Clear out the packaged high-glycemic foods you won't be eating any longer. Food banks welcome your contributions of canned goods and unopened pre-packaged foods.

As you continue to think "meat and vegetables" when you plan your meals, the concept will become second nature to you. And because you will be eating in alignment with the glycemic index weight-loss maintenance program for the rest of your life, meal planning and cooking will become easier and quicker.

Cooking Ahead

One of the glycemic index eating mishaps you want to avoid is arriving home very hungry and not having anything ready to eat. When you are very hungry, your body, mind, and entire being feel like you could devour a horse, but will settle for a loaf of bread or a box of crackers. You don't want this to happen.

When you arrive home very hungry and feel like you could eat a horse, first pause and drink a large glass of water. This is relaxing and will help get your mind working properly so you can quickly find some suitable food to eat. If you need to wait a few minutes for the food to heat up, make a cup of herbal tea to sip while you wait.

Keep a good supply of low-glycemic snack foods in your home, and we don't mean just celery sticks. We mean fruit, seeds and nuts, a variety of vegetables, and meats and fish. A great way to do this is to cook ahead and have the foods ready to eat when you walk in the door. Such meals as zucchini lasagna, fresh cut veggies, spaghetti squash with meat sauce, baked chicken breasts or drumsticks, barbecued pork ribs, or salmon salad can be waiting for you in the refrigerator.

> **Wrong Weigh**
>
> When selecting a low-glycemic or a low-carb cookbook, look for one that doesn't recommend the use of artificial sweeteners, especially aspartame. Or if the rest of the cookbook seems terrific, simply ignore the recipes that call for artificial sweeteners.

Cookbooks

Go to the bookstore and purchase three or four comprehensive low-carb and low-glycemic cookbooks. By comprehensive, we mean cookbooks that include useful recipes for breakfast, lunches, dinners, and snacks. You'll find suggested menus in Appendix D and recipes in Appendix E.

Read through them and get a feeling for the ingredients and preparation methods. Make a note of which recipes you and your family will enjoy. Then cook and serve. Yes, you'll be experimenting, but that's the only way to learn new life-supportive skills.

> **Body of Knowledge**
>
> Some cookbooks for persons with diabetes are based on the glycemic index and the recipes are positively scrumptious. Browse through this group of cookbooks when you're at the bookstore.

If anyone else in the family likes to cook, ask them to prepare a special low-glycemic meal for the whole family. That way, others can also take ownership for preparing and eating these delicious meals.

Cooking for Your Family

Preparing meals for more than one person can be challenging even without glycemic index eating as a factor. So let's look at some of the ways to manage and negotiate meals for a partnership or a family:

◆ Before you start on your glycemic index weight-loss program, call a family meeting to discuss your new eating needs and theirs. Ask for support and also assure your family that you'll be keeping their food needs in mind as you eat according to the glycemic index.

◆ Most important is that the basics remain the basics. Meat and vegetables should work for everyone. If you have an avowed vegetarian in the family, he or she can eat cheeses, eggs, seafood, and legumes.

◆ Practically speaking, other family members need to be able to eat their favorite foods—even if those foods don't fit in your glycemic index weight-loss plan. If you have the fortitude and strength, you can cook the family's favorite high-carbohydrate and high-glycemic foods. For example, cook biscuits made with wheat flour at the same time you cook ham and eggs for everyone. You can let others eat toast for breakfast while you enjoy eggs and fruit. If, on the other hand, you don't have the ability to avoid eating too much of the high-glycemic foods, you'll need to work out a different arrangement.

◆ There's nothing about low-glycemic foods or eating farm-sourced foods that will hurt anyone's health, so you don't need to apologize for the foods you prepare and eat.

◆ If your family demands high-glycemic snacks, assign a special place in the pantry for them. Just make sure you have a special place for low-glycemic treats, too.

◆ Prepare some whole-grain side dishes or "comfort food" recipes from low-carb and low-glycemic cookbooks to serve your family as well as yourself. You could find some real winners that please everyone.

◆ When the rest of your family wants to order takeout, such as pizza or Chinese food, order a salad or vegetables for yourself. Then you can eat the meat and vegetables from the food and pass on the pizza dough or sticky white rice. Basically, you can eat any takeout for a meal provided it contains protein such as meat or eggs, and you can fix a salad, fruit, vegetable, or low-glycemic whole grain as an accompaniment.

THIN-couragement

Meat and cheese rollups are simple and work for any meal or snack. Simply layer a piece of sliced meat with a slice of cheese and lettuce. Spread with mustard or mayonnaise. Roll up and secure with a toothpick. You can vary the meats, cheeses, and condiments according to your tastes.

Be patient and ask for patience from your family. Together you can work this out. There's always the real possibility that everyone's nutrition will improve because yours does.

Recipe Substitutions

You don't need to toss out your favorite cookie or cake recipes. You can modify them to be lower glycemic with great results most of the time. The recipes that work best are cookies, brownies, snack cakes, and quick breads, such as corn bread, muffins, or banana bread.

If you're up for experimentation, you could try these modifications for a layer cake, but we don't guarantee high and light results.

The two ingredients to modify are wheat flour and sugar.

Flour Substitutions

Based on how much flour the recipe calls for, use $^2/_3$ nut flour to $^1/_3$ Hi-Maize. Make nut flour by processing nuts in a food processor until you have flour. Nuts are highly nutritious and contain important good fats. When using nuts for baking, remember to keep your total fat intake for the day to 35 percent or less of total calories.

The best nuts to use are pecans, hazelnuts, and almonds because they're most reasonably priced and taste mild. You could try Brazil nuts and walnuts. Or, if your budget isn't a factor, try macadamias or pinion nuts. The conversion for processing nuts into flour is ¾ cup of whole nuts makes 1 cup nut flour.

You can also purchase nut flours in health-food stores and grocery stores.

Hi-Maize is a corn flour that's high in amylose, a resistant starch. Hi-Maize bakes like regular flour, has an imperceptible taste, and contains fiber that's health-promoting. Purchase online at www.amazon.com.

Sugar Substitutions

Table sugar is wonderful in baked goods: it has great taste, browns well, and is medium glycemic. Table sugar also satisfies your taste buds as no other sweetener can. Mixing it with a low-glycemic sugar like fructose or xylitol gives your baked goods great taste and lowers the glycemic value.

THIN-couragement

> Table sugar tastes great and cooks beautifully, but it's not a health food. It's medium glycemic but doesn't contain nutrients. Table sugar is a factory-sourced food but doesn't contain any mystery ingredients or questionably safe additives. Use it as a spice, rather than as the main course.

A low-glycemic natural sweetener is granulated fructose. A sugar alcohol is xylitol. Both of these taste sweeter than table sugar, so you can lower the amount you use by a couple tablespoons.

In your recipe, use half table sugar and half fructose, or use half table sugar and half xylitol. We prefer xylitol slightly, so find out which one you like best.

Wrong Weigh

> Honey is a wonderful food, but it isn't great for baking because it's a liquid and rather gooey/sticky. Baked goods with honey are sometimes too moist and chewy and never have that wonderful mouth feel of a regular cookie or muffin. Use honey in baked goods as a flavoring, but not as a sugar substitute.

Brown-Bagging It

You can pack any meal and take it to work, a meeting, or even your child's soccer game. Packing along food makes it easy for you to stay true to your glycemic index weight-loss program. Here are some sample menus for any time of day:

◆ If you aren't hungry for breakfast before you leave for work in the morning, pack breakfast. You can pack hard-boiled eggs, or meat and cheese rollups with low-glycemic foods such as farm-sourced plain yogurt, a small baked yam, cut vegetables, and fruit. If you have a microwave available at work, crack two eggs into a microwavable container and cover. When you're ready for breakfast, cook them in the microwave and eat. Add vegetables, a small amount of cold whole grains, basmati rice, or fruit as a side dish.

◆ For lunch or dinner, tote along any kind of main dish salad, such as a chef, Cobb, Caesar, or shrimp salad. Bring cold chicken or roast beef. Barbecued ribs work—provided you can wash your hands after eating. Add cut-up vegetables, low-glycemic whole-grain pasta, or fruit.

◆ For treats, pack some nuts, nut butters, olives, hard cheeses, moderate amounts (one third cup) of dried fruit, one or two pieces of fresh fruit, or larger amounts of cut-up vegetables. These are all reliably wholesome. The prepackaged tuna packs that contain tuna, mayonnaise, pickle relish, and crackers also work well for snacks. But hold the crackers and the candy mint—they're high glycemic.

◆ Don't be caught without snacks for long car trips, outings, and excursions where you might not be able to find suitable food. Be prepared and eat well.

◆ Bring purified water or herbal teas with you to events so you can avoid sodas and sweetened beverages.

◆ Take a packet or two of the electrolyte-balancing and energizing Emergen-C. Add to 8 ounces of water when you feel fatigued or stressed and need a quick, low-glycemic energy boost.

Taking along snacks and meals isn't just for people who are on a glycemic index weight-loss program. Many people bring snacks to work and to entertainment events because they prefer them to the factory-sourced high-sugar and high-glycemic snacks offered at ball games, festivals, and fairs.

The Least You Need to Know

◆ When planning and preparing meals based on the glycemic index, center them around protein and vegetables.

◆ Hold a family meeting when you begin your glycemic index weight-loss program to negotiate foods and family eating.

◆ Purchase some low-carb and low-glycemic cookbooks for meal and recipe ideas.

◆ Pack along low-glycemic meals and snacks when you're on the road.

◆ Modify your baked-goods recipes to make them low or medium glycemic.

Chapter 21

Special-Occasion Eating

In This Chapter

- ◆ Maneuvering special meals and emotions
- ◆ Eating at holiday meals
- ◆ Learning business-travel suggestions
- ◆ Vacationing the glycemic index way

When some people think of the holiday season, they immediately gain 5 to 10 pounds in their minds before Thanksgiving Day. Just thinking about special holiday cookies, candy, and breads seems to predispose people to weight gain. And for good reason—for many, the holidays aren't as much about gift-giving as they are about eating.

What's a person to do who eats based on the glycemic index during the holidays? Refusing a second helping of pumpkin pie from Aunt Judy may be viewed as a personal insult. Simply announcing that you're watching your weight is an invitation for other well-meaning family members to urge you to eat more. Plus, your declaration of intended weight loss is likely to elicit comments declaring that you look anorexic and malnourished.

The holidays are challenging times for people who eat mostly low-glycemic foods, as are weddings, vacations, parties, and public events such as street festivals and ball games. In this chapter, we guide you through the eating quandaries of all the special events in your life.

Your Inner Strength

Before we get into the details and specifics of eating at special events, you need to have an overall plan. Even people who have eaten unprocessed, lower-glycemic types of carbohydrates for years find it easy to slip up when eating at festive events that offer too many fancy cookies, cakes, breads, and candy. It isn't so much that they lack will-power or self-control, it's just that the total environment is permissive and disorienting. They get into the flow of the moment, and the flow simply isn't in alignment with mindful eating. Before they know it, they've eaten a funnel cake topped with chocolate ice cream and syrup and washed it down with a factory-sourced high-fructose corn syrup soda.

You've probably already experienced this, and you know how easy it is to get caught up in the frozen-chocolate-cheesecake-on-a stick mentality. Here's what it takes to enjoy an event without eating poorly in the junk-food or family-emotional flow:

- Stay conscious of your glycemic index weight-loss program. One of the joys of special events is that you enjoy time spent outside your usual life patterns. You get to have fun. But at the same time, you—as a person eating for glycemic index weight loss—need to remember your overall purpose in eating. That is, to eat more unprocessed, lower-glycemic carbohydrates, to continue losing weight, and then to maintain it.

- Ignore the fun junk foods. Cotton candy, Aunt Sara's fudge, blue sno-cones, Grandma's banana-nut bread, and candy Easter eggs hold fond memories from the past. That doesn't mean they'll light up your present if you eat them all. Eat selectively and mindfully. Ah, but those colored hard-boiled Easter eggs are low glycemic!!!

- Always sit down to eat when possible. No standing up or over the kitchen counter while eating.

- Don't overeat. Remember how awful you'll feel later if you overeat. You'll also feel awful later if you eat that factory-sourced junk food now.

- Assume that no one else will understand your food needs and that you have to take care of yourself. Unfortunately, this includes close family members as well as street-taco vendors.

- Focus on anything but food. Get in the flow of the event and not the flow of the food.

- Eat slowly and peacefully when you have the opportunity to eat low-glycemic foods. Think unprocessed, whole foods such as fish, poultry, meats, fruit, nuts and seeds, and vegetables at all eating opportunities.

- Keep a bottle or glass of purified water with you so you don't get thirsty.

- Both willpower and self-discipline are highly reliable for short bursts of time. Harness the energy of these personality strengths before the event so they endure for several hours at a time. Use them to avoid white, fluffy, or sticky high-glycemic foods and overeating.

- Enjoy and savor the low-glycemic foods at events—meat or seafood appetizers, fruit shish kebobs, deviled eggs, and other such foods.

- Don't let yourself get too tired, hungry, angry, or anxious. All these can trigger unnecessary eating.

Use all your internal resources to enjoy the special event. Learn to disassociate treat foods from specific events. In other words, hot dogs aren't a requirement for enjoying a ball game and pumpkin pie isn't going to make Thanksgiving any more complete.

Navigating the Holidays

You may be apprehensive about eating low-glycemic foods during the holidays and being faithful to your glycemic index weight-loss program. Your first low-glycemic holiday season is usually the most challenging. By the following year you'll know how to navigate the parties, family meals, and office treats with ease.

Holidays are times when you can enjoy these low-glycemic special foods:

- **Meats.** Roast turkey, smoked meats, baked ham, roasted pheasant, and game.

- **Fruit.** Some mail-order catalogs have beautiful fruit offerings.

- **Unshelled nuts.** These can be found along with fancy or plain nutcrackers in grocery and specialty stores.

- **Salted nuts.** Pecans, pistachios, and cashews, which can often be purchased from mail-order catalogs.

- **Unsweetened baked sweet potatoes and yams.** Eat in moderation, keeping in mind your daily carbohydrate allotment.

- **Imported specialty cheeses.** Both plain and smoked.

- **Vegetable trays.** Include nonstarchy vegetables such as celery, broccoli, cherry tomatoes, and cauliflower. Enjoy the good low-glycemic choices.

- **Specialty dark chocolates.** Enjoy and eat sparingly.

Be sure to take advantage of these wonderful low-glycemic holiday foods. Who says holiday foods are only about high-glycemic cuisine? Just be aware of the foods you need to avoid.

High-Glycemic Holiday Foods

The easiest way to deal with white, fluffy, and sticky holiday foods is to ignore them. They aren't going away, because many of those foods are part of our cultural heritage, but you don't need to eat them. Avoiding them isn't boring, it's wise.

Keep on thinking "meats and vegetables" when confronted with office goodies and family desserts, and learn to think differently about what the holidays mean.

It's easy for a person who loves food to focus on the eating aspects of the holidays, when, in fact, the holidays are far greater than the food. This year, focus on the people, the relationships, and your special religious observance. Think of the holidays as a time for good cheer and not just for good food.

THIN-couragement

Ask yourself how you can best celebrate the holidays. What special gifts can you give to others? These can be actual presents, but can also include gifts of time and caring for others in special ways. This lets you keep food and eating separate from the season's true meaning.

Family Traditions

Eating with your extended family for holiday meals can be either wonderfully supportive or oddly confusing. If your family truly supports your glycemic index weight-loss efforts, appreciate the situation. Eating with them will be easy.

If your family doesn't understand your weight-loss desires, you're not alone. Sticking to your glycemic index weight-loss program is challenging when important family members have contrary opinions. Here are some suggestions for eating with extended family:

◆ Avoid discussing your glycemic index weight-loss program. If anyone notices you've lost weight, say "Thanks" and change the subject.

◆ Eat protein and vegetables. Eat additional foods only as your weight-loss phase permits. In other words, avoid eating white, fluffy, or sticky foods.

◆ If anyone asks why you aren't eating as much as they want you to eat, smile and tell them you: a) aren't so hungry; b) are really enjoying the meats and vegetables; c) are more interested in their new projects, vacations, and so on.

◆ Ignore any off-the-wall or unkind comments about your size or weight-loss efforts and then change the subject. Keep possible discussion topics in mind so you don't miss a beat.

◆ Remember that you are neither anorexic nor malnourished. You're simply thinner than they remember. Thank them for noticing.

◆ If family members are truly supportive and interested in your weight-loss success, have fun discussing your program and answering their questions.

◆ Ask others plenty of questions about themselves.

As best you can in this potentially disorienting environment, keep in mind the true purpose of sharing holiday meals with family. Enjoy their company, feel the love, and stay in good cheer.

Wrong Weigh

You should ignore your family's concerns about your weight loss only if you are carefully watching that your BMI (Body Mass Index) doesn't drop below 19. If it does, your weight could be too low and you need to stop losing weight immediately. Being too thin is unhealthy and dangerous.

Parties

Parties are so much fun, especially when you don't need to deal with the food. Usually the food is great, but you know you can't eat as much as is presented on buffet tables. In fact, you may be getting dressed for the party while wondering how you're going to eat mostly low-glycemic foods amid a sea of cookies, cakes, and bread-based appetizers. Here's how:

◆ Don't start eating until you have reviewed all the food offerings. Zero in on the appealing low-glycemic foods and pass over any foods that don't look very appetizing.

◆ Talk to many people and put your energy into mingling and enjoying the people, not the food.

◆ Sip on club soda or mineral water with a twist, or empty a packet of Emergen-C into your soda. Add some ice and you have a vital, nonalcoholic energy replenishment.

◆ If you want a piece of wedding cake, have a taste. Ditto a sip of champagne.

◆ When appropriate, bring the hostess a gift of delicious low-glycemic appetizers, such as deviled eggs or sliced ham with fresh vegetables and condiments. Also add some acidic condiments such as dill pickles or marinated vegetables.

> **Wrong Weigh**
>
> Don't try to satisfy your sugar cravings with alcohol. If you choose to enjoy an alcoholic beverage, do as you would normally do. Don't increase your alcohol intake during the holiday season.

THIN**-couragement**

> Our favorite low-glycemic electrolyte replacement beverage comes in small packets that you add to water. The brand is Emergen-C and quite simply, there's no other product that comes close. It costs about 20 to 25 cents per packet. It's available at grocery stores and health-food stores. It replenishes you after exercise, stress, travel, sleepless nights—you name it. It contains vitamins, minerals, electrolytes, and no artificial ingredients. We wish we owned stock. Oh and yes, it tastes great.

If you are trying to come up with a fun idea for a party while staying on your low-glycemic plan, why not throw a mustard-tasting party? Simply purchase several different flavored mustards and serve them on cut-up vegetables such as jicama, celery, and carrots. Vegetables with enticing mustard makes a tangy snack that satisfies your need for crunchy and sour-tasting foods. The glycemic index is 0, with no fat. You can also hold a salsa-tasting party the same way.

On Vacation

Some people actually lose weight on vacations. They relax so much that their cortisol levels drop. They can then release built-up stored fat. Lucky them.

Other people gain weight on vacations. This is the situation for most people. But by eating wisely, you can continue your glycemic index weight-loss progress while on vacation. Here's how:

◆ Don't eat continental breakfasts—even when they're free—unless they offer meats, cheeses, fresh fruit, or eggs. Otherwise, you'll be eating free white, fluffy, or sticky high-glycemic foods. Instead, go to a restaurant for breakfast, or if you can, prepare breakfast yourself. You can also bring packages of tuna in your suitcase to complement the continental breakfast offerings.

◆ Keep your alcoholic beverage consumption the same as at home. Don't drink more than usual.

◆ Get enough sleep. Don't try to stay up too late every night, because your body could start to store more fat.

◆ Keep on thinking and eating proteins and vegetables.

◆ Don't go long periods of time without food or water. Plan to eat every four to six hours, or even more frequently depending on your body's specific needs.

◆ If you're in a foreign country with native cuisine quite unfamiliar to you, such as India or Thailand, bring along some familiar foods that you already enjoy, such as peanut butter, dried fruit, tuna, and shelled nuts.

THIN-couragement

Cruises offer plentiful food virtually all day and all night. Be selective in your food choices and don't get caught up in simply eating because the food is available. It's a superb opportunity to practice being discerning and picky. Take advantage of the plentiful exercise and excursion opportunities on board and off.

By following the previous guidelines, you'll be able to at least maintain your weight on the trip and quite possibly continue your weight loss.

Business Travel

Eating while traveling for business is challenging, especially when eating low glycemic. Any time your body's circadian rhythms are disrupted, your cravings for starchy foods increase because your blood sugar levels are erratic. Jet lag is a foe of dieters everywhere. But some simple guidelines can help you maintain steady weight loss with a business-travel lifestyle.

◆ Keep up your exercise program and stick to it faithfully. Fortunately, most hotels have exercise rooms and many offer fully equipped health clubs. Be sure you're up and at 'em early enough to take advantage of the fitness center. Pack your gym shoes and exercise clothes.

◆ Airline food is now nonexistent, unless you're traveling first class or very long distances. If you want to eat when flying coach, bring along your own food. You can purchase good main-dish salads from the airport concessions and also fresh fruit. If you have time, eat a sit-down meal at one of the airport restaurants, keeping in mind to order foods such as meats, chicken, fish, vegetables, and fruit.

◆ Pack foods and snacks for times when you won't be able to sit down and eat a meal. Bring along cans or packages of tuna, dried fruit, shelled nuts, natural beef jerky, a baggie of fresh-cut veggies, and cheese. Some hotel restaurants will provide boxed meals for breakfast, lunch, and dinner.

◆ At business dinners, continue to eat as recommended on your glycemic index weight-loss program. If you're famished, start with a low-glycemic appetizer and not with the bread basket.

◆ Because adequate sleep helps with weight loss, do your best to have a good night's sleep. If necessary, pack some creature comforts. Some people pack their favorite pillow, scented bath oil, music, or reading material to encourage a good night's sleep.

All the previous tips will help forestall an energy crash when your body's natural rhythms are out of sync—a fattening energy crash. If you have other favorite travel comforts, be sure to incorporate those into your business-travel plans.

At the Festival

Some special events offer up plenty of fun and plenty of fast food, but virtually no low-glycemic foods. We're talking about ball games, art festivals, jazz festivals, carnivals, state fairs, circuses, and many other enticing outdoor summer attractions.

You may be strolling along and all of a sudden the luscious aromas of waffle cones or the sight of freshly baked pretzels is too much to resist. What's a mostly low-glycemic eater to do? In addition to the enticing aromas, you'll see lots of people snacking and eating as they enjoy the full experience. You'll want to do the same thing.

Well, to put it bluntly, you can't take it all in. At least not the foods. You need some strategies:

- Find a food vendor that offers foods that are low glycemic. For example, a pulled-pork sandwich—hold the bun—with a side of vegetables is delicious and low glycemic. A grilled chicken sandwich works fine if you can forgo the white-bread bun. A chicken taco salad, hold the tortilla, is good low-glycemic fare. In addition to protein food and salads, corn-on-the-cob on a stick or fresh fruit might also be available at outdoor food vendors. Both of these are low glycemic.

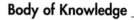

Body of Knowledge

Theaters offer the following treats as you sit watching a hilarious comedy or tear-jerking drama: pizza, french fries, popcorn, pretzels, and breadsticks. What could you order? Bottled water. Eat before you go to the theater and enjoy the show *sans* the white and fluffy foods.

- Stay away from the booths that offer the funnel cakes, popcorn, pretzels, and cinnamon rolls. Curiosity can easily kill a weight-loss plan.

- Keep bottled water close at hand.

- When you're hungry and want to eat a meal, find a restaurant, if possible, and sit down to eat.

- Don't get too hot and sweaty without electrolyte replenishment. Your body wants water and minerals, but your instincts could be to eat as a means of replenishment. Carry Emergen-C with you when you anticipate sweating in the hot sun.

THIN-couragement

Here's how to eat hot dogs or brats without the bun. You can use a fork and knife, but if that's too messy when eating on your lap, order the hot dog with the bun and your favorite condiments. Then, holding the bun in one hand, eat the end of the meat, and then slide the meat forward and eat the meat that's sticking out of the bun. Continue until all you're holding is the bun and the meat and condiments are all gone.

Taking action to prevent hunger and thirst frees up your energy to enjoy the fair or festival while you continue to lose weight down to your ideal size and then maintain it.

The Least You Need to Know

◆ You can find ways to eat low-glycemic foods at virtually any party or special event by eating meats, fresh fruits, and vegetables.

◆ Carry low-glycemic snacks on vacations and business travel for the times when low-glycemic foods aren't readily available.

◆ Gather your inner strength for sharing special meals with family and naysayers.

◆ At special events, focus your energy on the people and the purpose of the party and not on the food.

22

Quick and Easy Snacks and Treats

In This Chapter

- ◆ Finding quick low-glycemic snacks
- ◆ Packing along snacks
- ◆ Finding low-glycemic snacks almost anywhere
- ◆ Solving breakfast challenges

What do you do when you're hungry for something and you're not sure what it is? In the past, you may have scrounged through the pantry and refrigerator searching for that something that would satisfy your craving. Mostly likely it was a high-glycemic snack or even several of them—just what you didn't need.

While it's relatively easy to order a meal for glycemic index weight loss or to prepare one at home, it's generally more challenging to figure out what to eat for snacks.

In this chapter, we give you plenty of suggestions for low-glycemic snacks for home and other places. You'll find foods you can prepare and eat in and also some that you can carry with you when you are away from home.

What's in a Snack

Your ideal snack is easy to make or quick to find. But you need to be prepared for when a snack-attack hits. So fill your pantry and refrigerator with these low-glycemic treats for yourself and your family:

♦ **Stuffed dates.** Fill dates with ½ teaspoon of plain cream cheese or with an almond or pecan. Eating three or four gives you a glycemic load of 10. Any date lover will think "yummy!" Not familiar with dates? Start treating yourself!

♦ **Meat and cheese rollups.** Roll up a thin slice of meat and a slice of cheese in a lettuce leaf. Secure with a toothpick. Have one or two. There's no glycemic load. None! But there are calories in the form of protein and fat grams, so be sure to keep meat and cheese amounts within the limit for the day.

Body of Knowledge

Daily protein recommendations for the average woman by the American Dietetic Association are no more than 9 ounces of lean meat, poultry, fish, or an equivalent protein, and no more than 1 ounce of cheese per day. For men, it's no more than 12 ounces of lean meat, poultry, or fish and no more than 1 ounce of cheese per day. Equivalent protein foods include foods such as cottage cheese, eggs, and egg whites. A ¾-cup portion of cottage cheese equals the same amount of protein as 3 ounces of meat. Substitute two whole eggs for 3 ounces of meat.

♦ **Plain whole fruit with a cup of herbal tea.** Simple and delicious.

♦ **Snow-cones.** Although it's best to eat whole fruit rather than fruit juice, for a treat, make a snow-cone. Purchase a snow-cone maker at a kitchen store—they cost about $19.95. Fill the container that comes with the snow-cone maker about one third full with unsweetened juice or ¼ cup juice, top with water, and freeze. When you want a snow-cone, the snow-cone maker will churn out an icy treat in less than a minute. The glycemic load is about 3.

♦ **Pickled eggs.** You can find these at food specialty stores and at the deli. Make your own with the recipe for pickled eggs in *The Complete Idiot's Guide to Low-Carb Meals*. Even just one makes a filling snack. The glycemic load is 0.

♦ **Hard-boiled eggs.** They're an easy snack. Just keep a few in the refrigerator. The glycemic load is 0.

◆ **Cut up vegetables with dip.** For snacks, cut some vegetables into snack-size pieces when you arrive home from the grocery store. That way, they're ready for munching when the urge hits. When eating them raw isn't appealing, you can dip them in vinegar-and-oil salad dressing, a full-fatted dressing, or a lower-fat dressing. Try almond, cashew, or peanut butter, too. The glycemic load for all these is close to 0 per serving.

THIN -couragement

You can combine several of these suggestions into one snack. For example, you can eat a hard-boiled egg, a dried apricot, and one stone-ground low-glycemic cracker. Or enjoy a 1-ounce cube of cheese with a quarter slice of low-glycemic stone-ground bread.

◆ **Nuts or seeds.** You can choose from any kind of nuts or seeds you enjoy— macadamias, pecans, almonds, hazelnuts, pinions, walnuts, sunflower, pumpkin, and pistachios. You can eat them salted or spiced. You can find recipes for spiced nuts in many cookbooks. Just be sure that the topping doesn't contain sugar. Nuts and seeds by themselves have no glycemic load. Also be sure to measure out the amount of nuts you eat. It is easy to munch unconsciously and overeat. Eat slowly and you'll find that they become more satisfying and enjoyable.

◆ **Cashews and peanuts.** Although these nuts are low glycemic, they do contain a few more carbohydrates and thus have a slightly higher-glycemic load. Three tablespoons of cashews have a glycemic load of 3.

◆ **Parmesan crackers.** Picture a wafer of pure toasted Parmesan cheese. They're yummy and make a great party snack. You can make these ahead and enjoy them when you need a snack. Preheat your oven to 375 degrees. On a cookie sheet, spread one 6-ounce package of shredded Parmesan cheese into a thin layer. Make sure the Parmesan cheese doesn't contain potato starch or the crackers will burn and stick. Bake for about 10 to 12 minutes or until melted and slightly browned. Cool slightly, then remove the toasted Parmesan from the cookie sheet, and just break it into pieces. One or two pieces make a great anytime snack. The glycemic load is 0. A serving is 1 ounce.

◆ **Low-glycemic crackers and breads, such as pumpernickel rye kernel bread.** One ounce has a glycemic load of 6. Have one or two crackers or 1 ounce of bread. Suggestions for toppings include flavored mustard, a small slice of cheese, or 1 teaspoon of nut butter. Try tangy condiments such as chutney, olive tapenade, sun-dried tomato paste, or salsa.

◆ **Homemade trail mix of nuts, seeds, and dried fruits such as dried apricots and cranberries.** A serving size is 3 tablespoons. The glycemic load ranges from 1 to 2 when eating about ²/₃ nuts and seeds and ¹/₃ fruit. Eat small amounts—¼ cup or less—to keep calories and fat low.

◆ **Olives.** There are many varieties of delicious black olives or green olives. Eat three or four for a snack. The glycemic load is 0.

◆ **Cocktail onions.** Two or three make a nice snack. The glycemic load is 0.

◆ **Half of a small avocado.** Remove the pit and eat with a spoon. You can also fill the "hole" of the avocado half with salad dressing, such as vinegar and oil, Italian, or Ranch. Put the pit in the other half and wrap. The pit helps keep the avocado fresh. Place in the refrigerator and eat within a couple days.

◆ **Guacamole salad.** Prepare with ½ avocado, cut into cubes. Toss with lime juice, salt, and a sprinkle of chili powder. You can also add ¼ cup chopped tomato.

◆ **Sliced fruit such as apples, oranges, and pears.** One half of one of these fruits has an average glycemic load of 6.

◆ **Nut butters on fruit slices.** Use ½ tablespoon of peanut or almond butter on about 2 ounces of fresh fruit slices such as pears or apples. The glycemic load is about 2 to 3.

◆ **Beef or meat jerky.** Purchase jerky that doesn't contain mystery ingredients. You can find it at a natural-foods store or some specialty stores. (The convenience store varieties have enough chemicals in them to seem like you're back in chemistry class! Yuck.) Or make your own. The glycemic index is 0. As a bonus, jerky is low in fat.

◆ **Small cans of tuna or sardines.** Eat the tuna plain or mix with a small amount of mayonnaise. Purchase sardines in mustard or tomato sauce and eat right out of the can with a fork. When eaten plain, there's no glycemic load.

◆ **Dark chocolate.** Even a small square of chocolate makes a great snack. Rather than chew it, let the square dissolve slowly in your mouth. You'll derive great pleasure for a very low glycemic load of about 2. The antioxidants in dark chocolate are beneficial to your immune system and have been shown to help prevent skin cancer from the inside out.

◆ **Unsweetened fresh coconut.** A chunk or two makes for a fun snack for coconut lovers. There's no glycemic load, but it's surprisingly high in saturated fat.

- **Raw carrot sticks with fresh ginger and a cup of ginger tea.** The glycemic load is 3 for 1 cup of carrots or one medium carrot.

- **Small baked yam (½ cup).** Top with plain yogurt (2 tablespoons). Or sprinkle with cinnamon and 1 tsp. butter. The glycemic load is 7. Eat cold to increase the amount of resistant starch and lower the glycemic index and glycemic load to about 5.

- **Steamed fresh green beans (2 cups) lightly sprinkled with Parmesan cheese.** No glycemic load.

- **Hot blended green shake.** Cooked fresh beet or spinach greens with the cooked vegetable water, ½ ounce of feta cheese, and ¼ cup of cottage cheese. Mix in a blender after cooking for a warm revitalizing drink. Or drink chilled. This drink is filling and tastes great with no glycemic load!

- **Low-glycemic food bars.** Some food companies offer low-glycemic food bars. Check ingredients for mystery ingredients and artificial sweeteners.

- **Fruit frosties.** Put one cup frozen berries or fruit into a blender or food processor. Process until thick and eat with a spoon. Great for a summer cooler.

In addition to these snacks, go through the lists of low-glycemic foods in Appendix B and look for combinations that are appetizing and appealing to you. Always be sure that your snacks are within your daily glycemic load allotment.

Wrong Weigh

At the convenience store, you won't find low-glycemic treats on the candy shelves, inside the donut box, or nestled alongside the pretzels and chips. So don't even bother looking there. Why let yourself be tempted to blow your plans when you're tired, hot, hungry, and fatigued—in other words, desperate? In such situations, do the best you can. We've been there, too.

Herbal Teas and Beverages

Herbal teas offer wonderful tastes—earthy, exotic, comforting, summertime, holiday. Sample some and find your favorites. Some of our favorites are …

- Rooibos tea, also known as red tea. Originates in Africa. Contains more antioxidants than green tea. Tastes close to regular black tea, but without the astringent tang. Often packaged with other flavors. We prefer ours straight—iced or hot.

◆ Fennel seed tea. Add boiling water to a mug with 1–2 tsp. of fennel seeds. Use for digestion, especially a gassy tummy. Tastes mildly of licorice. Is already sweet tasting. Helps to reduce allergic reactions.

◆ Chamomile. A calming and soothing taste—great before bed or when stressed. An easy, gentle taste.

◆ Zinger teas by Celestial Seasonings. Choose a flavor you like from red to lemon. Sparkles in your mouth. Revitalizing.

◆ Ginger tea. Tastes slightly exotic and warming. Refreshing when served chilled. Use stevia for sweetening, if desired. Great for upset tummies and motion sickness, so sip during air or boat travel.

◆ Cinnamon tea. Herbal teas that contain cinnamon can help lower blood sugar levels and aid with glycemic index weight loss. Cinnamon is seldom the lonely ingredient in the tea, so look for a blend that contains cinnamon.

◆ Chinese regular and decaf green tea.

◆ Herbal Unwind-African honey bush with mandarin and orange.

THIN -couragement
> Research shows that women who drink at least 6 ounces of herbal tea a day have a lower risk of developing breast cancer.

Purchase herbal teas at the grocery and health-food stores. You can also purchase at tea shops and specialty stores. The very process of making a cup or mug of tea—putting the water on to boil, selecting your flavor, and then sitting down to enjoy the tea—is a calming and relaxing ritual.

Snacks on the Run

If you've ever tried to find low-glycemic snacks at a convenience store, undoubtedly you either walked out in frustration or you gave in and ate a white, fluffy, or sticky treat. Seems that convenience stores are little more than high-glycemic food filling stations. And the same holds true for the office snack machine and the snack counter at the movies. In this section, we give you some palatable suggestions for finding snacks at the most unlikely places.

◆ **Convenience stores.** If you're lucky, the convenience store has a bin full of fresh fruit, including apples or pears. If they don't have something fresh, you can probably find a snack of trail mix made with nuts, seeds, and dried fruit. You might find some suitable beef jerky. However, most brands of beef and meat jerky are filled with chemical preservatives and mystery ingredients, so read the labels carefully and choose the jerky with the fewest mystery ingredients. You may also find string cheese or unsweetened yogurt.

◆ **At the movies.** The snacks at movies are generally high glycemic. We can't recommend the candy, popcorn, or beverages. Most likely the best you can do is bottled water. Eat before you leave home. Better yet, bring a low-glycemic treat in your purse or coat pocket. (It really is okay, but unfortunately, some movie theaters police bringing in healthier snacks. So do what's appropriate.)

◆ **Lunch wagons.** Hopefully you'll find some fresh fruit and sandwiches and maybe pickled eggs or cheese. If the sandwiches are made with white or whole-wheat bread, you may need to hold the bread and eat the insides of the sandwich. Or only eat ½ piece of bread. Pickles and mustard are fine. Use lunch wagons as a last resort; instead, pack your lunch to take to work.

◆ **Office vending machines.** If the vending machines are stocked with only high-glycemic foods, you can petition the supplier for better food choices. Ask for small packets of nuts, trail mix, and fruit. Otherwise, steer clear of this part of the lunchroom and bring your own late-afternoon snack from home. Items such as dried fruit can be kept in your desk drawer for a long period without going bad.

Wrong Weigh

When the smell of office microwave popcorn wafts through the air at about 4 P.M., don't follow your instinctive urge to make a beeline for the lunch room. Popcorn is so high glycemic and the chemicals in microwaved popcorn are very factory sourced. Give yourself a break—breathe some fresh air, drink an Emergen-C or a big glass of purified water, stretch, and return to your tasks refreshed.

◆ **The coffee shop.** Perhaps you're meeting a friend for morning coffee or a late-afternoon latte, and you'd like a snack as well. Unfortunately, the snacks at coffee shops are usually baked goods made with white flour. They look scrumptious but are hardly low glycemic. Some coffee shops offer exquisite dark chocolate bars. You could purchase one and eat 1 or 2 squares.

◆ **At the ballpark.** Peanuts and crackerjacks are the trademarks of baseball games. Yes, enjoy the peanuts, but hold the crackerjacks—they're white and sticky. If you attend major or minor league sporting events, you already know the food doesn't

THIN-couragement

If you're planning an event or business meeting with a continental breakfast, consider asking the chef to offer hard-boiled eggs or some cold cuts of meats and cheese along with the standard fare. You'll find the meeting participants have more sustained energy and enthusiasm to carry them through to lunch.

fit in well with your glycemic index weight-loss program. Don't give up the ball games; instead, become very clever about the eating. Today, most ballparks don't let you bring in your own food. So you're stuck with the food concession offerings. Choose all-natural hot dogs, brats, or hamburgers, but forgo the bun. Purchase salads when you can find them. Pass on the sugary soft drinks, and instead buy bottled water or juice. Even though juice has questionable value, it does have some nutrition and you can limit the amount or dilute with water. A small glass of beer works if you're so inclined.

◆ **Continental breakfasts.** Continental breakfasts offer a wide assortment of all the wrong foods to eat for breakfast. Usually they are abundant with fluffy, white, or sticky foods such as Danish pastries, high-glycemic boxed breakfast cereals, and bagels. The butter, cream cheese, milk, juice, fruit, coffee, and tea are fine, but where's the food? What's missing is an adequate amount of protein: eggs, bacon, meat, cheese. If you are stuck eating at a skimpy continental breakfast, choose fruit and several packets of unsweetened cream cheese. This should hold you for an hour or two. It's best if you can pack along a couple snacks of hard cheese or a hard-boiled egg, or eat breakfast before you attend.

We predict that you'll find low-glycemic food offerings more widely available as soon as the popularity of eating based on the glycemic index grows. Until that time, be prepared. Carry along low-glycemic snacks to events, on airplanes, and to meetings. Keep some snacks in your glove compartment and your desk at the office. Follow the Boy Scout motto: be prepared.

The Least You Need to Know

◆ Keep low-glycemic snacks in your pantry and refrigerator for when you need a quick snack.

◆ Carry low-glycemic snacks with you so that you'll always have something on hand to eat.

◆ Eat discriminately at sporting events and the movies.

◆ Don't rely on convenience stores, coffee shops, and lunch wagons for low-glycemic food offerings.

Part 5

Insulin, Cortisol, and Weight Loss

Insulin and the stress hormone cortisol are metabolically connected, and they interact to affect your weight gain and weight loss. The less stress you have, the lower your insulin levels. The reverse is also true. The lower your insulin levels, the lower your stress.

When you learn to take action to reduce your stress on a daily basis and keep it lower, you'll find that losing weight, and especially losing weight through your waist and abdomen, is easier and, better yet, the weight stays off.

Chapter 23

Managing the Insulin/Stress Cycle

In This Chapter

- ◆ Understanding your body's stress cycle
- ◆ Knowing the role of cortisol in weight gain
- ◆ Avoiding cortisol-inducing foods
- ◆ Lowering your stress load

Let's say you have one of those weeks when your stress levels skyrocket. You face a major life-changing event. Your workload increases substantially although the hours in your week remain the same. Your energy levels were already taxed before dealing with normal, day-to-day stress puts you over your stress limit.

Then, at the end of the week, you step on the scales and find you have gained weight. Unfair! So unfair! After all, you were absolutely faithful to your glycemic index weight-loss eating program.

How can it be? What went wrong?

First of all, you didn't do anything wrong. Your glycemic index weight-loss program didn't fail you. Blame the stress. Stress all by itself can cause weight gain in everyone whether on a weight-loss program or not.

The reason is that your body's stress hormone, *cortisol*, plays a significant role in insulin function, which in turn can increase your weight. In this chapter, you learn how stress affects your insulin levels and how insulin affects your stress levels. The hormones cortisol and insulin play off each other and can make you a gainer or a loser, based on how cleverly you eat and manage your stress.

> **Glyco Lingo**
>
> **Cortisol** is a stress hormone secreted by the adrenal glands that stimulates the release of glycogen stores. Glycogen is the body's stored form of carbohydrate that changes into blood glucose in times of need. The extra blood glucose released when you're stressed increases stamina, endurance, and mental acuity when you need it most. Any extra is stored as fat.

Your Body's Stress Cycle

Stress just *is*. It is part of our lives, and it just isn't going away. Your body's response to stress is hard-wired directly into your biology to protect you. For instance, your body gives you a burst of energy when your safety is threatened. Your body's response to stress is actually very important to your well-being—that is, unless you live with chronic day-to-day stress and have no means of escape.

When stress becomes unrelenting, it can be seriously detrimental to your well-being. Too much ongoing stress can lead to heart disease, diabetes, depression, mood disorders, high anxiety, high blood pressure, autoimmune disorders, cancer, and other diseases and health disorders. Notice that these are the same chronic health conditions that can be caused by hyperinsulinism and insulin resistance (more on the similarities in a moment).

For now let's explore how your stress cycle works. The first phase is the excitation phase. This is triggered by an event that turns on your fight-or-flight response. The trigger event can be as simple as a loud and unexpected noise or the sudden news of a tight deadline at work. Your body secretes the stress hormones adrenaline and norepinephrine. It happens in a flash. Your heart pounds a bit faster, your reflexes become more sensitive, and subconsciously you become physically "on alert" to fight or to flee.

During the second phase, immediately after your body secretes adrenaline, your adrenal glands secrete the stress hormone cortisol. Think of cortisol as control central. Cortisol gives you stamina, energy, and courage, as well as the mental edge to make quick decisions and to resolve the situation. A high level of cortisol remains in your bloodstream until the stressful event comes to an end and you take time to decompress.

Body of Knowledge

Even our ancient ancestors experienced serious stress, but in general, they could decompress more easily because their stress triggers weren't as unrelenting as ours are today and because they exercised more. Imagine a caveman being chased by a wooly mammoth. His adrenaline starts pumping. He knows he has to take action or risk death. Cortisol kicks in and gives him the creativity, energy, and stamina to make a quick getaway and duck into a cave to hide. Scary, yes! But when the caveman is out of danger, his body begins to recover as he relaxes. The cortisol level in his body decreases. Although you and I might not want to live the lifestyle of a caveman, at least he had time to decompress! Many of us find ourselves in high-stress cortisol-inducing situations day in and day out. It's hard on the body.

After you have dealt with the stress, your body enters the third phase: the recovery phase. Your pulse rate returns to normal, the stress hormones are metabolized out of your body, and life calms down. In an ideal world, you cruise along easily until you encounter another big stress trigger.

In today's world, the three-phase stress cycle seldom has a clear beginning, middle, and end. Often a person doesn't decompress fully from one stressful event before another one starts. As a result, many people experience ongoing stress that never seems to stop.

They have many irons in the fire at one time, and their daily challenges keep on triggering more adrenaline and cortisol. They aren't pursuing ways like regular exercise to decrease stress. The levels of their stress hormones never return to resting. Instead, their cortisol levels stay elevated day after day and year after year, leading to weight gain, especially around the waist, and insulin resistance, metabolic syndrome, and eventually to chronic health disorders.

The Insulin/Stress Connection

The link between insulin and cortisol is parallel. When insulin levels rise, so do cortisol levels. When cortisol levels rise, so does insulin. In other words, chronically elevated insulin levels increase your stress levels. Stress increases cortisol, and the more cortisol in your body, the higher your insulin levels. Yes, this is a double bind. The question is how to step away from being a high-cortisol producing machine.

Insulin stimulates fat storage, glucose storage in the liver, and amino acid uptake by tissues. It's responsible for keeping your blood sugar levels within a narrow range.

But when you're under stress, you need your energy released from storage so that you can use it. Cortisol commands your body to increase blood glucose levels so it's available for the fight-or-flight event.

THIN -couragement

Public awareness and some of the scientific information about the intimate link between the levels of insulin and cortisol are relatively new. So stay tuned. As researchers dig further, they'll find more ways to help you manage your weight and your stress levels as the link between these two powerful hormones is better understood.

Cortisol commands your cells to stop uptaking sugar, which increases the insulin in your bloodstream. At that time, cortisol is directing your cells to become insulin-resistant.

Likewise, when your insulin levels are too high, the body will secrete cortisol. When a person is insulin-resistant, and has too much insulin in the bloodstream, the body secretes more cortisol to balance the effects of too much insulin.

In essence, your body's stress hormone, cortisol, causes weight gain. This is a fact of biology. What you can do to make this change is to keep your cortisol levels lower. We give you information and suggestions on how in this and the next chapter.

Cortisol-Inducing Foods

Overuse of some foods and medications causes your body's cortisol levels to increase. And guess what? Many of the foods are the same that directly increase your blood sugar levels, and ultimately, your body's insulin levels. Yes, including high-glycemic carbohydrates. Those foods are the following:

- Caffeine from beverages, such as coffee, sodas, black tea, and green tea. Especially beware the popular high-caffeine-powered sodas and energy drinks.

- High-glycemic starches and sugars. Avoid white, fluffy, and sticky foods.

- Beer, wine, and other alcoholic beverages.

- Too many grams of carbohydrates or too high a glycemic load eaten at one time.

- Caffeinated foods and beverages.

- Herbal stimulants, such as bitter orange and ephedra, which was banned for consumption by the FDA.

- Foods to which you are allergic or that you have a food sensitivity to.

- Allergic reactions to anything: trees, pollen, bug bites, food, petrochemicals, dust, mold, dander, and more.

Right now, you aren't eating high-glycemic starches and you're limiting your total carbohydrate intake, so you're already avoiding some foods that raise cortisol levels. But if you find that your weight loss seems to be stalled or that you're gaining weight, limit your consumption of caffeinated beverages and foods along with alcoholic beverages. Make sure that your exercise program is consistent and energetic.

It seems that everyone has a different tolerance level for cortisol-inducing foods. If you notice that a cup of coffee makes you jittery, hold the coffee and instead drink a beverage that's more soothing, such as an herbal tea or even hot water.

On the other hand, if a taste of chocolate within your carbohydrate levels is more soothing than enervating, go ahead and luxuriate in its taste. For some people, a little is fine, but too much puts them into cortisol overload.

Wrong Weigh

They don't call them beer bellies for no reason. Alcoholic beverages stimulate cortisol production, which leads to fat storage in the midsection—in the belly. This occurs whether the alcoholic beverage does or does not contain carbohydrates.

Weight-Loss Stress

Here's the rub: even the mere fact that you're on a glycemic index weight-loss program is stressful. You're trying to be more vigilant about everything you eat. You're making lifestyle changes, which produce more stress, even though they're positive changes. Even the foods you eat are different.

You're also monitoring your changes in weight, which is also stressful. Losing weight, being on a food plan, and dieting increase cortisol levels.

Yuck! Does this sound like you're caught in a vicious cycle? You're right. The cycle goes like this: the more stress, the more cortisol running through your body. The more cortisol, the harder it is to lose weight and the higher the possibility of insulin resistance. Insulin resistance causes weight gain.

But wait! There is a solution to this.

Other people have been highly successful losing weight on a glycemic index eating program, which means you can, too. The easiest way out of the vicious cycle is to accept that during your glycemic index weight-loss program, you'll have more stress initially, but that will subside after you eliminate stress triggers in other areas of your life. You also need to find time daily to reduce your cortisol levels through stress-soothing activities. We discuss those techniques in Chapter 24. After it becomes a habit to eat the glycemic way, your stress level will decrease.

It's not a good idea to start the glycemic index weight-loss program if you're in a phase of great stress. Wait until your life settles down before embarking on learning new ways to eat. In the meantime, eat carefully and avoid overeating.

Eliminating Stress Triggers

It's time to make a quick "stress analysis" of your life to figure out which stress triggers you can eliminate.

Certainly, many of your stressors can't be eliminated, but if you can let go of even a few, you may see immediate results as weight loss become easier. Here are some suggestions:

◆ Avoid rush-hour traffic on your way to and from work. Leave earlier or later to avoid high-stress traffic. For the long term, if you drive long distances to work every day, you may want to consider moving to a new location or finding a job that's closer to your home.

- ◆ If you're already stretched thin at work with an excessive workload, or at home with family responsibilities, say "no" when asked to take on more responsibility for outside activities, such as volunteer organizations or civic groups.

- ◆ If watching the news is distressing, especially right before bed, turn it off. Find other, more soothing things to do. Check out the stress soothers in Chapter 24.

- ◆ For the duration of your glycemic index weight-loss program, avoid making major life decisions such as marriage, divorce, job changes, increasing the size of your family, home remodeling, or other significant situations.

- ◆ Try meditation. Persons who consistently meditate at least once a day can find it easier to lose weight.

After you've eliminated as many stress triggers as possible, the stress triggers that remain are the ones you need to live with. But you can do something about them, too. That information is in the next chapter.

The Least You Need to Know

- ◆ When you're stressed, the stress hormone cortisol causes an increase in your body's insulin levels.

- ◆ Elevated levels of cortisol over time can lead to insulin resistance and weight gain.

- ◆ Too much insulin in your bloodstream can increase your stress levels by affecting your body's cortisol levels.

- ◆ Eating based on the glycemic index combined with stress reduction can increase weight loss and ease weight-loss maintenance.

- ◆ Exercise on a regular routine can help decrease cortisol and insulin levels.

Stress Soothers for Weight Loss

In This Chapter

- ◆ Preventing high cortisol and stress levels
- ◆ Decompressing from stress daily
- ◆ Finding a "crafty" way to de-stress
- ◆ Using cortisol-reducing supplements

Picture yourself coming home from work or another activity in the late afternoon or early evening. The day has been long and tiring, and your nerves are frayed. You search through the kitchen cabinets looking for a low-glycemic food—heck, any food!—that will mend your nerves. Nothing seems right.

But before you can relax, all the demands of the evening begin. You need to toss in a couple of loads of laundry, cook dinner, and then monitor the children's homework. You can't fathom finding time just for yourself. Even the notion of eating your dinner in a beautiful environment seems a remote luxury.

This situation is *not* conducive to weight loss, but what can you do? You don't need a pep talk about eating broccoli instead of cookies. You need a stress soother that reduces your cortisol levels, at least for the rest of the evening.

Don't despair! In this chapter, you discover many ways to reduce your cortisol levels and, simultaneously, reduce insulin levels so that you can more easily lose weight and maintain your weight loss. You'll be able to stop the vicious and fattening cortisol-insulin cycle.

Daily Anxiety Prevention Program

The best way to manage your stress is to control your body's stress response before it controls you. By using a spoonful of prevention, you can keep your cortisol levels lower all day long. You just need to follow a three-part program that's easy to manage. And it will be especially easy for you because you're already doing two of the three parts.

This cortisol-management program is great because it works for everyone. Trust us, it will work for you:

◆ Eat the low-glycemic way. Don't skip meals. When you eat carbohydrates, make sure they're low glycemic. Avoid starches unless they're low glycemic. By doing this, you're avoiding cortisol-inducing foods. Also, don't consume foods or beverages containing caffeine or alcohol. Avoid products containing bitter orange or other nervous system stimulants.

◆ Take at least 1 tablespoon of fish oil or cod-liver oil every day. The essential fatty acids in the oils help with brain function by regulating chemicals called prostaglandins. If these prostaglandins are disrupted, it causes anxiety, depression, and mood swings. Research shows that fish and flaxseed oils reduce symptoms of stress and soothe feelings of aggression and hostility. Plus, they aid in brain neurotransmitter functions. Research studies have been done on fish oil. Only fish oil contains *DHA* and *EPA*, which support neurotransmitter function. Fish oil and cod-liver oil are quite mild tasting and easy to swallow. You can opt for capsules or enteric-coated capsules if they're easier to take. Take five per day.

> **Glyco Lingo**
>
> **EPA,** eicosapentaenoic acid, and **DHA,** docosahexaenoic acid, are considered to be the most important omega-3 essential fatty acids. They are only found in animal products, especially deep-water fish such as salmon. They help rev up your fat-burning mechanism.

◆ Do vigorous aerobic exercise at least three times a week for 45 minutes. It will help get your heart rate up high enough for you to literally sweat. Sweating from exercise triggers the release of endorphins, your very own "feel good" chemicals. Taking a walk around the block doesn't work unless you walk or jog fast enough to work up a sweat. If you prefer, you can do vigorous sweaty aerobic exercise for 20 minutes every day. Vigorous exercise increases the flow of endorphins in your body and makes you feel good.

By following these three steps, you'll better handle the stress that comes your way. You'll be able to handle stressful situations without experiencing as much internal stress yourself.

Of course, some days and situations are harder than others. When confronted with new or more intense stress triggers, you'll still experience a rise in cortisol levels. That's why you need additional stress soothers to help you manage all the stressful events in your life.

Wrong Weigh

If you suffer from gallbladder or digestive problems related to fat metabolism, you may need to use only 1 teaspoon of oil or only a couple of the capsules initially and then see if you can gradually work up to more.

Decompress with Stress Soothers

Emily called herself high-strung. Unlike the motto "Don't sweat the small stuff," she did. She felt as if navigating life was like walking through a minefield. Her body size varied with her stress levels. Then she began eating the low-glycemic way and using the daily cortisol-management program. She was no longer on pins and needles after work. She could more easily handle the day-to-day chaos of raising a family and sustaining her marriage. Everyone involved breathed a big sigh of relief when she stopped sweating the small stuff ....

Some good news to remember: you can lower your cortisol levels without dramatically changing your life. You can improve your job performance, enjoy your family more, and have more fun. To do this, start incorporating stress reducers into your daily life.

Today researchers know what reduces stress because they can measure cortisol levels with a simple noninvasive saliva test. You might be a bit surprised by some of their results.

In one study, researchers tested the cortisol levels of a group of individuals. Then the test subjects hung out on the sofa to rest and relax. After an hour, the researchers retested the subjects and their cortisol levels hadn't changed. Seems sofa time is *not* a particularly good de-stressor.

They then had the same group do one hour of yoga. The cortisol retest showed a significant reduction in cortisol levels. Whoa! Yoga actually fulfilled its promise of soothing ragged nerves. What's interesting is that the very thing that a person would think of as relaxing—just lounging on the sofa—wasn't effective.

Here's a list of activities that are effective for reducing cortisol levels. Some may not suit your interests, but you'll find several that you can use regularly.

Get in Water

Warm water soothes your skin, which is the largest organ in your body. A warm-to-hot bath before dinner or before bed may be all you need to lower your cortisol levels and feel renewed. As you lie in the tub, imagine all your stress flowing from your body into the water and then down the drain. After your water break, put on some fresh clothes and enjoy the rest of the evening. If you bathe right before bed, snuggle into the covers and let yourself drift off to sleep.

You can get soothed in water in the hot tub, bathtub, shower, or even a swimming pool. Your immersion time can be very short. Even 5 to 10 minutes may be all you need.

You can make your bath more soothing and sensuous by adding bath salts, fragrant essential oils, or Epsom salts. Two all-time inexpensive favorites are sea salt and baking soda.

> **THIN-couragement**
>
> Getting hot also works for stress reduction. Regular Swedish saunas, steam rooms, and infrared saunas are a financial investment for your home. Their heat is rejuvenating, relaxing, and detoxifying. If you can handle the heat and the cost, sweat away your stress.

Get Some Sunshine

Experts tell us that our eyes need at least 15 minutes of sunshine or bright light every day for our hormones to function optimally and to keep our moods uplifted.

The best way to receive this blessing from the sun is to spend at least 15 minutes outdoors. Here are some simple options:

- Eat your lunch outside.

- Work in your garden.

- Take a walk.

You simply need to be in the sun without sunglasses for 15 minutes. Don't look directly at the sun. After 15 minutes, put on your sunglasses if you prefer wearing them.

THIN **-couragement**

> The interaction of the sun on your skin creates vitamin D₃, which is an important vitamin in helping prevent diabetes, autoimmune disorders, and cancers. For best vitamin D₃ production on your skin, you may want to put sunscreen on your face, but not on other exposed parts of your body unless you're staying out in the sun longer than 10 to 15 minutes. You can also obtain vitamin D₃ from nutritional supplements.

You may want to sit in front of a "light box" if the day is cloudy or overcast, or if you live in the northern part of the country where the sun doesn't shine much in the winter. These boxes are about the size of a laptop computer and they put out very bright light. Many people use them to remedy SAD: seasonal affective disorder. You can find one online by doing a keyword search for "light box."

Sunshine perks up your mood and helps you manage stress more easily.

Stretch Your Body

As you proceed through the day and your stress increases, your muscles tighten and contract. When you stretch, the muscles release the tension. This is one of the reasons yoga and other forms of stretching are so effective at reducing cortisol levels.

You can learn the correct ways to stretch by taking yoga classes or stretching classes. Or read one of the many stretching or yoga books available. *Stretching* is a classic stretching book by Bob Anderson. You can purchase DVDs on stretching at www. collagevideo.com. An Internet search will turn up lots of possibilities.

Stretch any time you need a refreshing break. You can stretch at the office, after your shower in the morning, after work, or right before dinner. Generally, it's easiest to stretch on an empty stomach.

The rules for stretching are quite simple:

- Be gentle. Don't force your body into a posture; instead, let your muscles open up to the stretch.

- Hold the postures until you feel your muscles release and relax.

- Go slow. Take your time. Stretching works best if you're moving slowly.

- Be patient. Over a period of several months, you'll be amazed at your new flexibility.

THIN-couragement

Stretching enthusiasts believe that as a person's body gains more strength, balance, and flexibility, those same qualities are incorporated into the person's life and way of being. Who couldn't use more internal balance, strength, and flexibility?

Stretching is also affordable. You really don't need any special equipment at all. Wear clothing that lets you stretch—either loose clothing or stretchy pants and tops designed for yoga. Consider purchasing a sticky mat that offers padding and prevents you from slipping. Beyond that, all you need to do is just do it!

Cross Crawls

This marching-style movement is amazingly helpful for stress and mental fatigue. March in place by lifting each knee high. When you do, touch the opposite hand or elbow to the knee. That's all you need to do for a minute or two.

The body-crossing motion of your hands and arms helps balance the right and left hemispheres of your brain while the light aerobic factor revs up your metabolism and endorphins.

Some health practitioners attribute other wonderful benefits to cross crawls, such as improving immune system function.

Personal Pamperings

Ahhh, those massages, facials, manicures, and pedicures. All of them can significantly reduce your cortisol levels. If you can afford them, by all means, pamper yourself and reduce your stress level at the same time. Some individuals find that a massage helps them stay stress-free for a week or two.

If you can't afford these spa-type treats, use the following personal pamperings that cost merely pennies per use or are totally free:

- **Find ways to trade pamperings with a friend or spouse.** For example, trade foot massages. Even 10 minutes of a foot massage goes a long way to relax you.

- **Use a back roller.** Check out the Maxi-Backsie at www.bodytools.com. It costs about $25 and lasts forever. And it's highly relaxing. A back roller looks like a wooden rolling pin but with waves in it. To start, place it just below your neck. As you relax, your body weight will help the tool work deep into the erector muscles along the spine. Then slowly roll down your back while the tool moves with you. Take about 5 to 10 deep breaths at each vertebra. By the time you reach the lowest part of your back—after about 15 minutes— you'll be wonderfully relaxed. The back roller relaxes the erector muscles on either side of your spine and massages acupressure points and lymph glands along the way. Use the back roller anytime you need to de-stress. There is also a smaller one to use for traveling or when sitting down.

> THIN-couragement
>
> The back roller is also known as the Ma Roller. Benefits attributed to its use read like a health tonic: it massages acupressure points for organs and glands, moves lymph fluid from lymph glands that are located along the spine, helps detoxify the body, and realigns the spine. It's a wonderful process, and you may find still other benefits that you enjoy.

- **Use a still-point inducer.** You can find one online at www.gaiam.com. It costs about $25 and lasts forever (like the back roller). Just lie down with your upper neck-lower scalp on the inducer. Lie still for 5 to 10 minutes and let the inducer's gentle pressure create the "still point," a quiet pause in the rhythm of the craniosacral system. Users claim many beneficial and therapeutic effects as well as deep relaxation. Some people prefer to listen to soothing music while using the still-point inducer, but it works wonderfully when used in silence.

- **Try body rolling.** Find information about this highly relaxing method of body alignment at www.yamunabodyrolling.com. Body rolling uses balls ranging in size from a couple inches to about 8 inches in diameter. Spend a half hour rolling down your thighs, up your back, or on your feet and you'll feel great. Body rolling is used for body realignment, because it works somewhat like deep-tissue massage or structural integration. We think it helps eliminate cellulite and flatten puffy tummies. The cost for the beginner kit is $59.

With a little imagination, you'll discover many other forms of personal pampering. When you find one that works, use it often to lower your cortisol levels and keep your mood calm and even.

Brush Your Hair

It almost seems too simple to be true: brushing your hair is both relaxing and good for you. Many women—and men—have intuitively known this for years. Brushing your hair helps get your stress hormones back in balance. The best hairbrush to use is a very inexpensive one that has plain plastic bristles that are rough on the tips, which stimulate your scalp better. The hairbrushes with rounded plastic tips may not work as well.

To brush your hair, bend over from the waist and brush, making sure that the bristles are reaching through your hair to your scalp. Brush for a minute or two, then stand up and rearrange your hair. You'll feel great—refreshed and energized.

You can brush your hair anywhere that you have a brush and a private area. Yes, restrooms work just fine for this.

Dry Brush Your Body

Purchase a natural-bristle brush made specifically for dry body brushing. They're stocked at health-food stores and some discount chains.

Preferably before your morning shower, brush your body when it's dry. Start with your feet and work up your legs and torso toward your heart. Then brush arms, shoulders, and upper torso.

This is highly invigorating. Brush very gently. You'll be exfoliating dead skin cells and the motion of the brushing helps move lymph fluid to detoxify the body. It makes your skin smooth and strong. But most of all it makes you feel good and uplifts your moods.

Arts, Crafts, and Hobbies

Hobbies are healthy. Well, at least most of them are. An activity that shifts you out of work mode, or life-maintenance mode, into a world of creativity, rhythm, or beauty will help you tackle everyday stress. The hobby that you enjoyed as a young person may be the same one that brings you relaxation and a sense of serenity today. Of course, the list of possibilities is endless, but here are some ideas for getting started:

◆ Handicrafts, such as knitting, crochet, needlepoint, sewing, or quilting.

◆ Visual arts, such as sketching, painting, photography, sculpture, scrapbooking, or pottery.

◆ Gardening or flower arranging.

◆ Woodworking, home repair, rebuilding cars.

◆ Playing a musical instrument.

◆ Writing letters, poems, novels, articles, and journal or blog entries.

◆ Puzzles, such as crossword puzzles, jigsaw puzzles, and Sudoku.

◆ Leisurely reading.

◆ Games, such as bridge, Scrabble, and Monopoly.

◆ For some people, cleaning, ironing, or house-painting are stress soothers.

It seems amazing that so many highly enjoyable activities reduce your cortisol levels. But don't get out of control with your hobby. Yes, you can be productive and also reduce your stress levels, but don't let your fun activity create more stress.

In other words, do your arts, crafts, and hobbies as leisure activities and not with deadlines and urgency. Don't let your hobbies consume you—they'll only create more stress.

Meditation and Prayer

Many persons have had huge success with reducing cortisol levels through a process known as "stilling the mind." Research studies show that individuals who meditate regularly, meaning once or twice a day, experience better sleep, lowered blood pressure, and decreased risk of cardiovascular disease and stroke.

If you are interested in pursuing meditation or prayer as a means to reduce stress, you have many choices. For centuries, people have used prayer, contemplative prayer, and meditation. The basic technique for meditation is to sit still for 20 minutes twice a day, preferably morning and late afternoon. The meditator focuses on a mantra, which is a series of simple syllables, and repeats the mantra aloud or silently while breathing in and out. That's all there is to it. It sounds simple, but it can create profound calm. Contemplative prayer offers the same benefits.

You can learn to meditate on your own by using a meditation tape or DVD, or by simply reading a book on meditation and doing the suggested exercises. Or you can take a meditation class. Many classes are offered through extension centers at universities and community colleges. You can also take courses on prayer and contemplative prayer through your church or place of worship.

Stress-Soothing Supplements

Recently some nutritional supplements have been shown to reduce cortisol, and they've been finding their way to health-food store shelves. So check them out and, if they work for you, use them either daily or when you're feeling highly stressed.

Some of these supplements are advertised as helping with weight loss. They can be a partial answer to avoiding insulin resistance and the ensuing weight gain, but they aren't the total answer for attaining one's ideal size.

◆ Green tea contains compounds, especially theanine, that are calming. If you can handle the caffeine in the tea, you can drink as many as three cups a day. If the tea hypes you up, you need another choice.

Wrong Weigh

Before you stock up on cortisol-reducing supplements, be sure you're taking the basic nutritional supplements recommended in Chapter 16. Many of them, such as the B vitamins, calcium, and magnesium, provide you with the extra nutrients you need when stressed.

Use caution when taking these cortisol-lowering nutritional supplements. While they're readily available at health-food stores, you may want to consult with your health practitioner before you use them. Some may work well for you and others won't. Record when you use these in your food diary and also write down any positive or negative results. That way, you can find the combinations that work best for you.

◆ Theanine as a supplement can help control stress. It's an amino acid found in green tea leaves, but you can purchase it in capsules at any health-food store. Theanine relaxes you without sedating you. In fact, theanine helps increase your brain's production of alpha waves, the brain waves associated with alert thinking and reasoning. No known adverse side effects have been reported. You can use theanine daily or when needed, but don't take more than 200 mg per day. You'll feel its effects within a half hour and the relaxation lasts for about two hours. We don't recommend that you take theanine before bed, because it increases your mental alertness and to sleep you need to turn off your active brain.

◆ Epimedium is an herb that comes from an ornamental bush grown in Asia and the Mediterranean. In research studies, epimedium extract reduced blood levels of cortisol and improved immune system function. Be sure to purchase water-extracted epimedium, because it has shown no adverse side effects. You can use up to 1,000 mg per day for cortisol control.

◆ Phytosterols are found in fruits, vegetables, nuts, and seeds. You're already enjoying their benefits when you eat two to three servings a meal. They modulate your immune function, reduce inflammation and pain, and help control allergies. They also reduce cortisol levels. You can purchase phytosterols as a supplement, but we encourage you to get all or most of these phytosterols from food. If you do want to take a supplement, take between 100 and 300 mg per day of a mixed phytosterol blend that includes beta-sitosterol.

◆ Magnolia bark helps control cortisol levels and is beneficial for lowering anxiety and stress. However, if you take too much, you could experience drowsiness or sedation. Some minor side effects have been reported, but it's generally considered safe. Purchase magnolia bark to prepare as a tea or in pill form. You can take between 250 and 750 mg per day.

◆ 5-HTP (5-hydroxytryptophan) is a form of one of the essential amino acids, tryptophan. Tryptophan converts in the brain into serotonin, which can help improve mood, decrease appetite, and improve sleep. Initially start with a small dose (30 to 50 mg) on an empty stomach, preferably in the late afternoon or before dinner. Don't take 5-HTP with food because it's not effective then.

Read the label carefully. Some of the supplements can be taken regularly, up to three times a day. Others may work best when used on an as-needed basis. And don't use all the previous supplements at the same time—that's way too much. Start with one and determine if it works for you. If not, try another one. Stop if you have any negative reactions. Hopefully, you'll find one or two that work well for you.

You can find stress formulations at health-food stores that combine several of the previous supplements into one pill. You'll need to experiment to find a formula or product that works best for you (see Appendix C).

Wrong Weigh

Don't use 5-HTP every day, but rather use it once every other day or about three times a week. Taking the supplement too often can cause some of the same side effects as the SSRI antidepressant medications. These include Prozac and Zoloft.

The science of cortisol-control through supplementation is new, and you can expect more news and more supplement formulations as research progresses. As more people use these for cortisol control, expect more reported side effects and more information on how they work in the body. Before you use any of these supplements, do further research on the Internet to read about possible side effects and usage recommendations.

Weight-Loss Supplements

You've read the ads and watched the infomercials about the latest weight-loss supplements. Perhaps you've tried them but down deep in your heart wondered if they are effective, and perhaps more importantly, safe to use.

They're probably safe when taken only in the recommended amounts. Probably they don't work as well as you'd want. If they did, they'd be major headline news.

If you're still curious, ask the company selling the weight-loss supplements to send you follow-up photos of the before-and-after pictures. Request photos of those men and women one year after their terrific weight loss. Of course, you'll never receive them. They would have regained all the weight and more. It's because that kind of quick weight loss brings with it a rebound effect. Always.

The Least You Need to Know

- Use the daily anxiety management program to keep cortisol and insulin levels low.

- Take time daily to decompress and relax using one of the stress soothers.

- Develop a fun interest in arts, crafts, or hobbies that will help you manage stress and lower your cortisol levels.

- Cortisol-reducing supplements work to chemically reduce your cortisol levels and assist with weight loss.

Chapter 25

Toxins and Glycemic Index Weight Loss

In This Chapter

◆ Releasing toxins

◆ Avoiding an increase in toxins

◆ Learning the detoxifying functions of the liver

◆ Using the glycemic index to reduce toxins

◆ Managing your body burden

Most people cringe when they learn their bodies are filled with toxins. Just the thought that more than 100 toxic chemicals are present in the average person's body seems … well … it seems unbelievable. But that's not all. Those toxins can block your body's ability to release stored fat.

A person with a higher toxin load has a more difficult time losing weight. Fortunately, a glycemic index weight-loss program helps the body release toxins and promotes eating healthful farm-sourced foods. Farm-sourced foods usually contain fewer toxins than factory-sourced foods.

In this chapter, you learn how toxins play a role in weight loss and how low-glycemic eating helps you release the toxins that normally tend to prevent weight loss.

Your Toxin Load

We all have *toxins* in our body. There's nothing anyone can do to avoid getting at least some toxins inside the body. We acquire toxins from the foods we eat and the air we breathe. Toxins are absorbed through the skin from skin lotions, sunscreens, and household cleaners.

> **Glyco Lingo** _____
>
> **Toxins** are chemical substances that harm or irritate the body. They may contribute to inflammation and chronic health disorders. A person breathes in toxins from air pollution and petrochemical fumes and consumes them when eating or drinking, taking medications, and through skin contact with some cosmetics and cleaning products.

Toxins can be either water soluble or fat soluble. Water-soluble toxins are stored in water-based body fluids, such as lymph fluid and blood. Fat-soluble toxins are stored in body fat.

By storing the toxins away from major body organs, your body is protecting you from being poisoned. Actually, this is rather ingenuous when you think about it. But losing body fat reduces your body's toxin-storage capacity.

Toxins Stored in Fat

As your body uses stored fat for energy when you lose weight, the toxins that were stored in body fat are released into your bloodstream, tissues, and organs. Because toxins are poisons, this sudden flooding can make you feel awful. You can feel irritable or experience headaches, nausea, and lightheadedness.

Do you recall how you felt during the first couple weeks of a previous weight-loss program? Most likely, you didn't feel all that great. If you're like most dieters, you attributed that run-down feeling to being deprived of the foods you loved. Certainly that could have been the reason for feelings of emotional deprivation. But in truth, toxins were flooding your system and making you feel under the weather.

Major sources of toxins include the following:

◆ Environmental pollution that you breathe, including car exhaust and gasoline fumes

◆ Secondhand smoke

◆ Medications, including over-the-counter medications

◆ Poor-quality drinking water

◆ Plastic water bottles that leach bisphenol A (BPA), which is most of them

◆ Pesticides, herbicides, fertilizers

◆ Steroids and growth hormones used for meat, fish, poultry, and milk production

◆ Paint, carpet, and household cleaner fumes

◆ Many skin creams and topical ointments, such as bug spray and sunscreens

◆ Perfumes, nail polish, and acrylic nails

◆ Cosmetics and hair products

◆ Most factory-sourced foods

◆ Aspartame, also known as Equal

◆ Food additives such as artificial colorings, flavorings, and preservatives

> **Wrong Weigh** _____
>
> Some health experts believe that too many toxins in the body lead to more fat storage. They hypothesize that the body will actually conserve fat and create even more fat in which to store the toxins rather than let the person be poisoned.

You can't avoid all the previous sources, but you can minimize your exposure to them. If you're a woman, of course you're going to wear mascara and lipstick. So minimize the toxins when you can. When you do, you lighten what's known as your *body burden*, the amount of toxins that your body has to deal with.

> **Glyco Lingo** _____
>
> **Body burden** denotes the amount of toxins that an individual has within their body at any point in time. A high body burden of toxins has been indicated as the cause of serious disease conditions such as cancers and autoimmune diseases. As you ease your body burden and help promote toxin flushing from your body, you may experience important health benefits.

The Liver as a Detoxifier

Your liver is the organ that manages two important functions as you lose weight. When you eat a low-glycemic diet, your liver converts stored fat into energy. This is what makes glycemic index weight loss so effective. Your body uses stored fat for energy rather than glucose from carbs. You want your liver to be in tip-top condition to perform this important function efficiently.

The second function of the liver is to process out body toxins. All toxins go through the liver on their way out of the body. Toxins can be eliminated through sweat, urine, feces, breath, and mucus. But they don't get there until they first go through the liver.

The liver works based on priorities. First it processes out toxins, and then it converts fat to energy. If its workload of toxins is too high, it may not get to its lower-priority jobs, such as converting fat into energy so you can lose weight. Yes, that means you won't lose weight as fast.

It's to your benefit to reduce your body burden and keep it low so that you can lose weight faster and more efficiently. Do this by avoiding the following foods and beverages:

◆ **Alcohol.** You've heard that drinking too much alcohol over a lifetime can destroy liver function through a disease called cirrhosis of the liver. What you may not know is that even a drink or two takes energy away from your weight-loss efforts because the liver's top priority is to detoxify all alcohol a person drinks

◆ **Chemical food additives.** These are the kinds you are avoiding on your glycemic index eating program by eating mostly farm-sourced foods. These include food colorings, preservatives, and artificial sweeteners. Avoid foods that contain these "mystery" ingredients.

◆ **Caffeinated drinks.** Too much caffeine from such foods and beverages as coffee, black or green tea, kola nut, guarana, chocolate, cocoa, colas, and some over-the-counter pain medications, in addition to affecting cortisol levels, prevents proper hydration, thus making it harder for the liver to eliminate the toxins. If you drink a moderate amount of coffee—two to three cups or caffeinated soft drinks a day—don't be concerned. But if you drink more than that, consider cutting back. Drink plenty of plain purified water to support liver function.

◆ **Sugars.** To efficiently metabolize calories, the body needs nutrient-dense foods. Empty calories cause stress on the body.

◆ **Diets low in fiber.** When you eat for glycemic index weight loss, you are eating plenty of fiber. Don't ever return to a low-fiber diet. You need 25 to 45 grams of fiber a day. High-fiber diets help the body remove toxins from the digestive tract faster.

◆ **Too much animal fat.** Toxins are stored in animal fat, just like in human fat. Be sure to cut excess fat from meats, poultry, and fish before eating.

As you can see, by eating low-glycemic foods you are actually helping your liver convert stored fat into energy because you're lowering your body burden.

Body of Knowledge

To avoid the PCBs and other toxins in oceangoing fish, purchase fish that's harvested farther out into the ocean and not close to shore, such as farm-raised fish. To prevent consuming mercury found in oceangoing fish, avoid swordfish, shark, and king mackerel, and limit canned tuna to one serving twice a week.

Removing Toxins

The previous recommendations help you avoid adding to your body burden by avoiding the sources of toxins. But you can go even further and actually reduce your body burden by supporting your liver in functioning well and by accelerating the process of flushing toxins from your body. To do this, follow these tips:

◆ **Eat plenty of vegetables and fruits.** Veggies and fruits contain antioxidants, which neutralize the free-radical damage that can be caused by toxins. They also include plenty of fiber, which helps move toxins from the body through the bowels. Aim for 25 to 50 grams of fiber a day and two to three servings of vegetables and fruits per meal.

◆ **Eat mostly farm-sourced foods and avoid highly processed foods and junk foods.** Generally speaking, these contain a lot of toxins. Read the ingredient list and you'll find food colorings, chemical preservatives, and plenty of ingredients that are impossible to pronounce. If you assume that many of the unpronounceable ingredients contain toxins, you'll be right about 80 percent of the time.

◆ **Eat essential fatty acids in your foods and take an essential fatty acid supplement in the form of fish oil daily.** These good fats help remove toxins from the body. Purchase your fish oil supplement from a reputable company.

◆ **Drink lots of purified water every day.** Water flushes out water-soluble toxins and also the fat-soluble toxins that have been converted by the liver to water-soluble ones. The tried-and-true recommendation to drink eight glasses of water a day may be overdoing it. That's too much for some people and not enough for others. If you live in a dry, hot climate, you may need more. If you live in a humid area, you'll need less. Drink enough water so you don't get thirsty or dehydrated. Only water qualifies as water. Other liquids are beverages.

Body of Knowledge

People who are overweight and obese are usually dehydrated compared to people of normal weight. A person's body composition is made up of body fat, muscle mass, and water. When body fat is high—over 30 percent—a person has less water percentage. This makes it harder to lose weight. Remedy this by enjoying an electrolyte beverage such as Emergen-C daily and drinking more water than you think you need. Avoid electrolyte beverages that contain ingredients and additives such as maltodextrins, corn syrup, artificial flavoring, coloring, sweeteners, and preservatives.

◆ **Exercise.** Exercise is wonderful for supporting all metabolic functions, including the liver's function. Exercise lets you sweat out the toxins. A couple of great ways to move lymph are doing jumping jacks and bouncing, as on a mini-trampoline. Bouncing stimulates movement of lymph fluid, which carries toxins from the body. They're fast ways to detox and fun exercises. If you're new to these exercises, though, take it slow. You don't want to overload your system and get the flu or a cold.

◆ **Stretching.** As you stretch, you mobilize toxins to go to the liver from muscle and fat to be processed from the body. Stretching is time well spent.

◆ **Massage.** Ask a message therapist to give you a lymph-detoxification massage. The lymph nodes found all over your body are the gathering place for toxins. The lymph system doesn't have a pump, like the cardiovascular system does. What moves lymph to the liver is your physical activity: exercise, stretching, dry brushing, and lymph node massage. The back roller massages lymph nodes along the spine.

◆ **Sweating.** Use the sauna, infrared sauna, or sweat lodge to remove toxins through the skin. This is one of the reasons that sweating feels so good – you're refreshed in many ways.

◆ **Supplements.** Take antioxidant nutritional supplements to go along with your antioxidant-rich vegetables, fruits, and herbal teas. Toxic substances trigger inflammatory prostaglandins. Antioxidants help protect against the free radicals that occur due to this inflammatory process.

To avoid the run-down feeling when toxins are being flushed from your stored fat, be sure to follow the previous recommendations during your entire glycemic index weight-loss program.

Obviously, avoiding unnecessary toxins is a good lifelong endeavor for general health. Toxins add unnecessary and unwanted stress on your body. Because you'll be eating based on the glycemic index indefinitely *and* avoiding toxins, you'll get a double benefit: a great-looking body and a healthier one, too.

THIN-couragement

Find out if your cosmetics, skin care, hair care, or perfumes contain toxins at www.cosmeticdatabase.com. You can check out pet products at www. petsfortheenvironment.org. Some skin-care companies put only safe ingredients in their products, so you have many options today, and many companies are actively removing toxins from their cosmetics and skin-care lines.

The Least You Need to Know

◆ Toxins are stored in body fat and are released when a person loses stored fat through weight loss.

◆ During weight loss, the released toxins can cause headaches, irritability, and fatigue.

◆ As best you can, avoid increasing your body burden or toxin load by making lifestyle changes.

◆ By following a glycemic index weight-loss program *and* avoiding toxins, you can lose weight and boost your overall health.

◆ Take positive action to help your body release toxins through exercise, diet, and using products that don't contain known toxins.

Part 6

The Exercise Advantage

Exercise for weight loss isn't about burning calories and body fat. Those intentions can put you on an endless anxiety-provoking treadmill to keep the weight off. You don't need to work that hard or that intensely to lose weight.

The physiological and emotional benefits of exercise to your body's biology are far more significant. Use aerobic conditioning, strength training, and stretching or flexibility training. They enhance your body's ability to reduce emotional eating, release toxins, shape and tone, improve digestion, and increase muscle. The resultant increase in metabolism and well-being is your reward.

Exercise becomes the ultimate health tonic and one that's economical—it hardly costs you anything.

Chapter 26

Give Your Body Movement

In This Chapter

◆ Using aerobic exercise

◆ Reducing insulin resistance

◆ Creating an aerobic conditioning program

◆ Improving moods and ending emotional eating

Movement is our word for exercise. Don't think of long hours spent huffing and sweating at the gym with before-and-after trips to the scales. That's boring and not sustainable. After all, who has long hours to spend at the health club? Or even wants to?

Movement is a life essential. It's a free health and weight-loss supplement. It cures most of what ails you and improves what it can't cure. So what's not to like about exercise?

All the excuses. It makes you sweat, you need a shower and shampoo after, it makes you uncomfortable, you don't have time, you're lazy, you have better things to do, it interrupts your daily life (which is probably a good thing), you'd rather read a good book, and so on. You're creative and you can think of some great reasons not to exercise.

But if moderate and consistent exercise could keep you thin for life, could you find a way to exercise for at least 20 minutes up to a full hour a day? We're sure you could, and in this chapter we'll begin to show you how.

Aerobic Exercise

The first type of exercise your body hungers for is aerobic exercise. This form of exercise is now often referred to as cardio, which is short for *cardiovascular.* Whatever you choose to call it, you need moderate *aerobic exercise* for at least 30 minutes, 5 times a week or vigorous-intensity aerobic exercise for at least 20 minutes 3 times a week. By the end of the 20 minutes, you should be sweating. Okay, women are supposed to glow and the guys sweat. Call it whatever you choose, but be sure to do it.

Running, jogging, swimming, and bicycling are popular forms of aerobics as are vigorous hiking, racquetball, tennis, dancing, and aerobic conditioning classes. Add in winter sports like cross-country skiing, snowshoeing, and ice skating. Golf, bowling, fishing, and billiards are pastimes and are not in any way considered aerobic activities.

> **Glyco Lingo**
>
> **Aerobic exercise** is exercise that you do for a sustained amount of time, at least 20 minutes, that moves your major muscles such as thighs or arms and makes you huff and puff and break into a sweat.

Perhaps you've read or heard that heavy housework and gardening are adequate substitutes for aerobic exercise. They are, but only if you do them constantly for over 15 minutes and work up a sweat. (Make sure the sweat isn't due to a high outdoor temperature in the garden, but because you have exerted yourself.) For most people, housework and gardening aren't adequately aerobic. So do your housework or gardening, but be sure to add a regular aerobic exercise routine.

Aerobics and Insulin Resistance

Aerobic exercise is an important activity in supporting your weight-loss program. The biological benefits enhance the health benefits of the glycemic index. Vigorous aerobic exercise increases your cells' ability to uptake glucose. This is important if you have insulin resistance, hyperinsulinism, or diabetes.

Here's why: in all the above conditions, the body's cells refuse to obey insulin's commands to uptake glucose. This means that too much insulin stays in the bloodstream and that blood glucose levels are too high.

Elevated levels of insulin and glucose mean that your body stores the glucose as fat and you gain weight. Insulin resistance can also lead to metabolic syndrome and diabetes.

When you do aerobic exercise, you actually improve the entire insulin-glucose-carbohydrate cycle, making it more efficient. Although this mechanism doesn't sound like it's about losing weight, it is. The ultimate result of reducing or eliminating insulin resistance is that your body uses insulin and glucose efficiently. You have more energy and less fat storage.

When your insulin levels are balanced, so is your level of the stress hormone cortisol, meaning that aerobic conditioning reduces stress—both long-term and short-term.

Just reading this information may inspire you to lace up your shoes and start moving. But wait, there are still more weight-loss benefits to cardio exercise, so read on.

THIN-couragement _____

If you feel sluggish or fatigued, or if you are bombarded with carb cravings, aerobic exercise may be the answer. Even a couple of minutes can perk up your metabolism and energy levels and energize your cells, because they'll be getting an extra boost of glucose. If you eat carbohydrates when you're sluggish, fatigued, or plagued with cravings, you could experience weight gain and lowered energy levels while increasing the cravings. The answer: when you crave carbs, do some exercise.

Aerobics and Fat

Aerobic exercise burns fat. It takes energy—namely calories—to fuel your body. During aerobic exercise you burn through plenty of calories. When you're eating for glycemic index weight loss, your body also burns stored fat for fuel. So you get a double boost when eating low glycemic.

The primary sources of fuel for aerobics are carbohydrates and fat. At the start of your aerobic exercise session, your body uses glycogen stores (your body's form of carbohydrate) for fuel. After those are used up, the body uses fat.

Wrong Weigh _____

Can a person exercise too much? It's theoretically possible, but unlikely. A solid hour a day is plenty. Don't overdo it, though, or you could have aching, tired muscles that keep you laid up for a few days. If you are a triathlete or marathoner or if you exercise vigorously for more than one hour a day, you need to eat more carbohydrates to maintain strength and stamina.

If a person is eating a higher-carbohydrate diet, the body doesn't use as much fat as its fuel source. An added bonus of an exercise program: the more trained a muscle is, the greater its ability to use fat as fuel. Exercising regularly and consistently increases your fat-burning capacity. The result is that it's easier to stay at your ideal size.

The length of time of your exercise sessions pays off. Any amount of aerobic exercise burns fat, but of course, the longer you exercise, the more fat you burn.

Don't worry, you don't need to turn into a gym junkie to burn more fat. Just an extra five minutes a day can make a difference.

Aerobics and Your Protein Needs

People who are athletic generally need to eat slightly more protein to maintain strong muscles. The same holds true when you're losing weight. The protein guidelines in this book account for your increased need: about 3 to 4 ounces three times a day.

Aerobics and Your Heart

When a person has insulin resistance, the excess insulin causes the body to store fat initially as triglycerides. Yes, these are the same triglycerides that contribute to high levels of LDL—the so-called bad cholesterol. It's the type that clogs arteries.

When you do aerobic exercise, you reduce insulin resistance, thus reducing triglyceride storage. At the same time, you increase your body's good cholesterol, called the HDL level. The HDL, or high-density lipoprotein, helps carry away excess cholesterol.

That's the first piece of good news. But there's more. Aerobic exercise strengthens your heart muscle and its pumping efficiency. Aerobic exercise is a gift to your heart. And because your heart is the core of your body, it's a gift you give to yourself.

Aerobics and Your Moods

You've heard about the runner's high, which happens when endorphins are released and bring on uplifted, energized, and happy feelings. Low levels of the brain neurotransmitter serotonin and others can lead to feelings of depression, anxiety, and carbohydrate cravings.

You can use aerobic exercise to boost your moods. Many formerly depressed people say it's the best drug there is. Exercise increases the feel-good brain chemicals that override carb cravings and emotional overeating. Yes, this is all totally legal, widely available, and better yet—free.

THIN-couragement

> Doing exercise is free but it could cost you to get started. The cost may be a onetime cost: running shoes, hiking shoes, flex bands, exercise ball, stationary bike, or treadmill. You can spend more money to stay fit by joining a fitness center or paying for lessons, but you don't need to. You can always tune into exercise shows on TV and work along for free.

Aerobics and You

By now you are excited about the upside of aerobic exercise and are facing the same challenges that everyone ever devoted to a sedentary lifestyle faces. You can only reap the rewards if you physically start to move.

First of all, you have to, absolutely have to, ignore your own objections, complaints, justifications, and excuses. And you need to adopt the best exercise slogan ever written—Nike's "Just do it."

Then you need to decide what you're going to do. Here are some of your choices:

◆ **Stationary bike.** We love this because we can read while we pedal away for 20 minutes in the morning. Plus, if you purchase a stationary bike, you can exercise at home. You can also watch television while pedaling. Be sure you don't get so involved in your reading or program that you slack off on pedaling with vigor. Stationary bikes are great if you have weak or damaged knees that limit your ability to jog or use the treadmill.

◆ **Jogging or running.** If you like to jog or run, go for it. Start slowly and then increase your weekly mileage by no more than 10 percent per week to prevent injuries. Your basic equipment is nothing more than a good pair of running shoes, socks, sunscreen, and a sun-protective hat.

◆ **Swimming.** Make sure you like getting wet and then find a pool, lake,

Body of Knowledge

Before you embark on a new exercise program, especially if you are out-of-shape and unaccustomed to exercise, check with your doctor. Also, if you start experiencing excessive pain or fatigue, seek professional health care and advice.

or ocean. Other than a body of water, all you need is a swimsuit and perhaps goggles and a swim cap. Swimming is great if you're just beginning to exercise or if you have lots of aches and pains that could preclude high-impact exercise.

◆ **Cardio machines.** These include elliptical trainers, treadmills, stationary bikes, and stair-steppers. Most fitness centers offer these along with a television to help you while away your vigorous aerobic minutes.

◆ **Walking.** Choose walking only if you're just beginning to do aerobic exercise. You'll benefit initially because you'll be moving. But after several months, you'll need to pick up the pace to continue receiving benefits. The best way to walk is to make sure that your heart rate is at the correct level for your age (discussed in the next section). Strolling isn't the same as walking. Think quick, brisk, fast, huff, and puff. Soon your walking can turn into taking hills at a brisk clip.

Wrong Weigh

Avoid the stair-stepper if you were born with larger or shorter thighs. Instead of making them thinner, you could actually increase both their strength and size. Instead, choose another type of aerobic exercise. Intense stretching exercises could help make them feel longer and look smaller. We talk more about stretching in Chapter 28.

◆ **Aerobic classes.** Offered at fitness centers, these classes are designed to keep your heart rate up for at least 45 minutes to an hour. Not only will you be moving to the music, you'll be gaining strength from calisthenics and other exercises. Be sure to attend class two or three times a week. You'll find many variations of aerobic classes, ranging from African dance to cardio yoga.

◆ **At-home videos.** You'll find a wide variety of aerobics DVDs and videos online at www.collagevideo.com. These are a great choice if you like to exercise at home. They're very convenient and excellent for bad-weather days and travel.

◆ **Racquet sports.** Do you enjoy racquetball, squash, or tennis? These games are excellent for aerobic conditioning when you play with vigor and competitiveness. But if you prefer to talk through the game and take it easy, find another way to get your heart rate up.

◆ **Outdoor aerobics.** If you love the great outdoors, you can do your aerobic conditioning outside. Hiking, mountain biking, snowshoeing, and cross-country skiing are all excellent for aerobic conditioning.

◆ **Contact sports.** If you love basketball, volleyball, football, soccer, and other contact sports, go for it. These sports require skill, agility, and a certain toughness. Be sure you develop the required toughness before you play intensely. You absolutely don't want to be sidelined with injuries. Aerobic conditioning is supposed to be fun.

◆ **Other gym equipment.** Yes, you can use other types of gym equipment for your cardio exercise. Just be sure to elevate your heart rate for a minimum of 20 minutes a day or more.

Mix and match your aerobics. You could hike for two to three hours on the weekend, attend an aerobics class on Monday after work, and pedal on your stationary bike at home in the mornings before work. No matter how you combine your activities, do at least 20 minutes a day or more.

Your Heart Rate

Now that you're enjoying aerobics, you're technically an athlete. As such, you need to be concerned about the quality of your conditioning. It only makes sense that you want to exercise in the best way possible.

In aerobic conditioning, your heart rate counts. Here are guidelines for your target heart rate zone for your age.

Age	Target Heart Rate Zone at 50%-85% maximum heart rate	Maximum
20	100–170 beats per minute	200
30	95–162 beats per minute	195
40	90–153 beats per minute	180
50	85–145 beats per minute	170
60	80–136 beats per minute	160
70	75–128 beats per minute	150

While you're exercising, take your pulse to determine your heart rate. Some machines give you a real-time readout of your pulse rate. If you don't have an electronic readout, here's how to take your pulse:

1. Find your pulse on the inside of your wrist or at the side of your neck just below and in front of your ear.

2. Wear a watch with a second hand. Count your pulses for six seconds and multiply by ten. That's your heart rate. If you want to be more precise, you could count your pulses for ten seconds and multiply by six. In either case, you get close, and that's all you need. If this doesn't appeal to you, you can purchase a heart monitor from a sporting goods company and use that.

Wrong Weigh _____

You don't need to ease up on your aerobic exercise program as you start your glycemic index weight-loss program. Don't sit at home instead of exercising. Suit up and show up even if you don't want to exercise. Most likely you'll do some movement and immediately feel better about going.

In the midst of your aerobic session, your heart rate needs to be near the moderate number or above it. That means your heart is working hard enough. It's fine if your heart rate is higher than that, but don't exceed the maximum for your age unless you are in great shape.

This is what you need to know: if your heart rate isn't high enough, your aerobic training isn't doing you much good. Yes, working out properly means you'll huff and puff and that you'll sweat.

However, if you can't catch your breath, slow down. Check your heart rate and make sure it isn't too high based on the preceding chart. For the best results, keep your heart rate at a level where you can still talk while exercising.

Aerobic Do's and Don'ts

Use these guidelines as you embark on your aerobic training. Success and pleasure breed more success and pleasure, and we want both for you. Because you'll be participating in aerobic conditioning for the rest of your life, here are some ways to boost your success quotient:

THIN-couragement _____

If you have the time to watch even one television show a day, you have time to exercise. Place your stationary bike in the TV room and pedal along to your favorite show. Many gyms now have exercise machines with their own TVs.

◆ Start slow. Build up your endurance as quickly as you can without overdoing it. If you're new to exercise, you need some time and patience to acclimate.

◆ If you're new to exercise and you have a family history of heart disease, high blood pressure, impaired glucose tolerance or diabetes, or if you smoke cigarettes, consult with your health practitioner before beginning your program.

◆ Wear comfortable shoes and clothing. Blisters or sunburn will sideline you, and they aren't fun. If your feet are blister-prone, wear two pairs of thin socks when you exercise. If you can predict the location of potential blisters, put a Band-Aid on the spot before you put on your socks and shoes. And always break in your athletic shoes before a big event or pack along a second pair just in case.

◆ If you glow rather than full-out drip sweat, you may not need a shower after exercise. On the other hand, if you do sweat, you need to make plans for a shower afterward unless you plan to spend the rest of the day in isolation.

◆ Beware of infomercial exercise products. Some work. Some don't. If you make a purchase, be sure you can return the product if you're not satisfied with your results. Also beware: you simply can't achieve satisfying aerobic, strength, flexibility, and health results in 5 or 10 minutes a day. So avoid gadgets that tout fitness in mere minutes a day.

◆ Beware of fitness club January specials unless you actually plan to use the club year-round. Be sure to check out your total financial commitment before you sign on the dotted line.

◆ Plan aerobic fitness strategies for rainy days, days when you don't have a car, and days when you're on vacation or out of town. Fortunately, most hotels have fitness facilities and the rooms have DVD players for exercise videos.

◆ Exercise with a friend. This keeps both of you motivated and more likely to exercise and not skip planned sessions.

◆ Think of exercise as an indulgence rather than as a chore. Everyone needs pampering and a way to let off steam. Although exercise is really a life requirement, think of it as a luxury. That way, you're more likely to indulge.

◆ Keep your body hydrated. Bring along packets of Emergen-C along with bottled water. Use if and when you need to replenish your electrolytes.

◆ When you feel like you're going to boil over with stress, let off some steam through exercise – aerobic, stretching, or even just a walk.

◆ Regardless of whether you want to exercise or not, get dressed and show up. Failing to show up means that you could eventually give up, and you don't want to do that.

◆ Get to know your body—its capabilities and its limits. That way, you'll be doing the best aerobic training that meets your body's needs.

- If something in your body starts hurting, stop exercising. Find out what's wrong and correct it before you start up again.

- When you start out, don't give in to your competitive urges. Instead, work at your own pace until you're ready to show off. Be sure to exercise within your heart rate range.

As you continue your aerobic conditioning, you'll discover new things about yourself and your inner strength. You'll leave the naysayers behind and establish a reliable conditioning program for yourself.

Adaptation and Progress

As you continue to exercise, your body will become accustomed to the amount and intensity of your aerobic conditioning. In other words, your aerobic exercise will become easy. This is good because you've achieved a new level of fitness. But it also means that your body is ready for more.

It's time to up the intensity or length of your workout, or both. If you're using a stationary bike, increase the resistance, pedal faster, or pedal for an additional five minutes. If you're swimming, go faster. Hike up steeper hills or take longer hikes. If you're walking, go faster or move up to speed walking. Increase the incline on your treadmill. Your body wants you to do this, so give your body exactly what it wants.

Aerobic conditioning actually pays you. Over time, you'll be paid with less fat, no insulin resistance, a stronger heart, and lower stress levels. All you need is to "just do it."

The Least You Need to Know

- Aerobic exercise increases the cells' uptake of glucose and reduces insulin resistance and metabolic resistance while helping you lose weight.

- Your body requires at least 20 minutes of aerobic exercise daily, and more is better.

- Aerobic exercise burns fat and elevates your mood.

- Find several types of aerobic exercise that you enjoy and can do in a wide variety of circumstances.

27

Boost Metabolism with Strength Training

In This Chapter

◆ Boosting your metabolism

◆ Lowering your body fat percentage

◆ Learning how to train for strength

◆ Doing the five Tibetan exercises daily

What have you always wanted your body to look like? Certainly you want your body to be at its ideal size and to stay at that size for life. But beyond size and weight, how do you want your body to look?

Imagine yourself in a swimsuit at the beach. Most likely you want your muscles to be lean and toned. Certainly you want your upper arms to appear strong and tight rather than wobbly and wiggly. You can't achieve these things through what you eat, although what you eat definitely helps. You can only achieve a body that approximates your ideal through strength training.

In this chapter, you learn the very real advantages of strength training to boost your metabolism, help you lose weight, and keep it off. You learn how to make your muscles strong and buff. As a bonus, you'll learn about a simple morning exercise that boosts and balances metabolism and more—the five Tibetans.

Benefits of Strength Training

Strength training, also known as resistance training, gives your muscles shape and definition. It also gives you many weight-loss benefits.

Avoid Weight-Loss Sagging

You're concerned about how you're going to look after you've lost the weight. You could end up with sags and bags, or you could end up lean and buff. If your body shrinks in size as you lose weight without the skin surface area also "shrinking," you could end up with loose skin hanging down from your upper arms, waist, stomach, and other areas. By the time you attain your ideal size, the only solution for tightening up your skin is plastic surgery. The surgeon cuts away the excess skin and sews the edges together. This is uncomfortable and expensive, and leaves scars. This kind of drastic sagging skin situation usually occurs when a person has more than 75 to 100 pounds to lose. But even if you have less weight to lose, you could end up with sagging skin and skin folds.

You can avoid sagging skin by starting to do something about it today. Start strength training now and continue throughout your glycemic index weight-loss program and beyond as you maintain your new size. That way, your skin will shrink along with the rest of you. By the time you attain your ideal size, new people you meet will have no idea that you were ever overweight. Why? Because your skin will fit your body.

Strength Training and Metabolic Resistance

Metabolic resistance means that a person's body is resistant to weight loss. This comes from years of yo-yo dieting and going into and out of starvation metabolism, which leads to high body fat percentage.

The basic rule of metabolic activity is this: the higher a person's body fat, the slower his or her metabolism, and the harder it is to lose weight. The lower a person's body fat percentage, the higher his or her metabolism, and the easier it is to lose weight and to maintain it.

One of the fastest ways to reduce your body-fat percentage, and metabolic resistance to weight loss, is with strength training. Dietary protein also helps boost your metabolism. To assure your success, be sure to eat 3 daily servings of high-quality protein— 3 ounces 3 times a day for women, 4 ounces 3 times a day for men. You'll love the fast results you'll achieve.

THIN-couragement

Judy's body fat was 38 percent and it seemed that no matter how much she ate or what she ate, she couldn't lose weight and keep it off. Then she started attending two one-hour Pilates classes a week. Pilates is a form of strength training that includes stretching. Within six months, her body fat was down to 28 percent and she was losing weight with less effort. She was wearing a smaller size and her muscles looked more toned and solid.

Here's a rundown on what affects metabolism:

◆ **Age.** The younger a person, the higher his or her metabolism. As people age, their metabolism slows down. Older bodies require less food to stay thin. The body's hormone production slows with age, and the body stores more fat.

◆ **Hormones.** The lower a person's hormonal production, the lower his or her metabolic rate. This includes estrogen, thyroid, testosterone, and progesterone.

◆ **Body fat.** A person with high body fat has a slower metabolism.

◆ **Eating high-glycemic carbohydrates often will lower your metabolic rate.** Eating low-glycemic and higher-fiber carbohydrates can increase your metabolism by helping you maintain your muscle mass.

◆ **All forms of exercise.** Exercise can increase your metabolic rate. The amount of time invested and the intensity of the exercise influences how much your metabolism is increased. But if you overdo the exercise and strictly cut calories, your metabolism goes into starvation mode and slows down. So do enough exercise, but don't overdo it.

Obviously, there's nothing you can do about your age. And although some research shows you can boost hormone production through exercise and activity, as far as anyone knows to date, you can't really turn back the hormonal clock; you can only delay its progress.

Wrong Weigh _____

Julia had already lost 30 pounds, but still had 40 pounds to go. She attributed her weight loss to eating low-glycemic foods and getting plenty of exercise. When her body hit a plateau, she increased the duration and intensity of her workouts at the recommendation of her trainer. Pretty soon, she was spending two to three hours a day at the fitness center and was still on a weight-loss plateau. Julia was overtraining. By cutting back her exercise routine to about one hour a day, her body can get back in balance and start releasing stored fat again.

However, you can make changes with regard to your body fat and your eating. After you begin to master eating low-glycemic carbohydrates, the next step is to master your body fat percentage.

THIN -couragement _____

The U.S. government recommendation for exercise is, as of this writing, set at one hour a day for optimal health and fitness. The hour can be cumulative from several activities you do during the day. If you can't fit in one hour every day, can you do seven hours a week?

Getting Thinner, Weighing More

To understand how body fat percentage works, your body is composed of three things: fat, muscle, and water. A person's water percentage ranges between about 50 percent to 60 percent.

The rest is made up of muscle or fat. It's the balance between muscle and fat that determines the portion of your weight that you have healthy control over.

Here's a chart that shows the recommended body fat percentage range for men and women by age.

Women:	
Up to age 20	14–21 percent
Age 20 to 50	17–27 percent
Age 50+	20–30 percent

Men:	
Up to age 20	9–15 percent
Age 20 to 50	14–21 percent
Age 50+	19–23 percent

If your body fat percentage is within the range for your age, you won't be flabby. In fact, you won't be overweight. But you could actually weigh more than you think you should. Don't despair. This could be highly beneficial.

Two people who appear to be the same size and height could have very different weights. The person with a higher muscle mass will weigh more because muscle weighs more than fat. For example, suppose a woman who is 5'5" wants to weigh 125 pounds and wear a size 8. If she increases her muscle mass through strength training while she's losing weight on a glycemic index eating plan, she could get down to her desired size 8 and weigh 135 or even 140. But there's no reason for her to panic or be disappointed in herself. She's wearing the size she wants to wear. Her body measurements are what she wanted. Her muscles look great—so what if she weighs more than her original goal?

)┤I┃(-couragement

> People don't know how much you weigh, they only know how you look and how your clothes fit. How much you weigh is your personal business.

Wrong Weigh

Lean people have a higher percentage of water in their bodies; people who are overweight have a lower water percentage, which means they could be continually dehydrated. This prevents weight loss. Be sure you're drinking enough water every day. Also, to keep your body's water percentage high, you can supplement with electrolytes. Avoid drinking commercial electrolyte beverages that are high-level factory-sourced and contain high-fructose corn syrup or artificial sweeteners. Instead, take electrolyte tablets or use a powdered drink mix such as Emergen-C.

This could happen to you, too, as you do strength training. What you weigh is less important than the size of your body. The entire situation is healthy, provided that your body fat doesn't drop below the minimum in the previous charts.

Set body fat percentage goals and clothing size goals as well as weight goals. Body fat percentage and clothing size are far more important than your weight goals because they're what truly tell you how you look and give you a better indication of your overall health.

THIN -couragement

As you increase your muscle mass, you may want to go beyond your original goal of increasing metabolism along with basic toning and shaping. You could decide to take up muscle building as a hobby and intentionally bulk up. In that case, you need to train longer and harder with increasingly more resistance, so check out personal instruction with a well-qualified professional who is certified by a respectable association such as ACSM, NSCA, or ACE.

Stamina, Energy, and Strength Training

Muscle gives you a performance advantage. Muscles give you stamina and endurance—not just for exercise, but for all your activities. More muscle gives you the ability to keep going when the going gets tough. You'll have more energy to do the activities you love, more energy to keep up with your children and work activities, and more ability to stay on your glycemic index weight-loss program.

Look Smaller Now

You want quick results, and you can achieve them with strength training. After only three months of two hour-long strength-training sessions a week, your body will become smaller. Your waist will be smaller, as will your upper arms, and your stomach will be flatter.

It will seem like everything pulls in closer to your bones, because muscle takes about $^2/_3$ less space than fat. Combining glycemic index weight loss with strength training is a surefire way to lose weight and look smaller within weeks.

Getting Started

You only need two sessions of strength training a week. If you feel really ambitious, you can do three, but don't do any more than that. Strength training causes small tears in the fibers of your muscles. This is good, because as the muscles repair on your "off" days, they become stronger and tighter. If you do strength training every day, your muscles won't have time to rebuild between sessions.

Schedule each session for 45 minutes to an hour long. Here are some equipment choices you can use for strength-training exercises:

- **Free weights.** Very popular, easy to use, widely available. Start with two- to three-pound weights and add weight as your body adapts. You'll know when this happens because the exercises will become too easy and your muscles won't fatigue during a session.

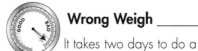

Wrong Weigh

It takes two days to do a strength-training session. On the first day, you lift weights or work with resistance for 45 minutes to one hour. On the second day, you rest and let your muscles recover and heal. Then, about 48 hours after the first session, you can do another one.

- **Stretch tubing.** A stretchy thin tube with handles on each end. Resembles a jump rope. You can purchase them in several levels of resistance—green, blue, red, and black. Great when traveling.

- **Flex band.** A long, wide, stretchy band used for resistance training. Great for traveling.

- **Ankle and wrist weights.** Strap them on for resistance as you do strengthening exercises. Don't run or jog with ankle or wrist weights, because you could seriously hurt your ankles and knees.

- **Body bar.** A long, weighted bar used for resistance training. May or may not have additional removable weights on either end.

- **Fitball.** A big inflated ball on which to do exercises. This ball looks innocent enough, but just wait until you do crunches and sit-ups and more with the ball. It provides a highly challenging strength-training workout.

- **Magic circle.** A circular handheld ring, about 15 inches in diameter with handles across from each other. By compressing the circle with legs, arms, and other body parts, you can get quite a workout.

- **Pilates classes and equipment.** Pilates is an exercise method that creates lean, flexible, and strong muscles, plus very strong abs and terrific posture. Pilates is a core-conditioning type of exercise.

- **Exercise machines** at fitness centers. You can set the resistance of the machines to match your strength levels. They can also be purchased for home use.

◆ **Power-pump classes.** An exercise class where you lift weights and move to the beat. Fun, and the energy of the group makes the time pass quickly.

There are many variations of each type of equipment and exercise. As you can see, you have plenty of choices for developing your own strength-training program.

$\int\!\!\!\!\int\!\!\!\!\int\!\!\!\!\int\!\!\!\!\int$ -couragement _____

> Not all strength-training approaches work for everyone. If you dread picking up free weights, a Pilates class may be exactly the right approach for you. You can vary your form of strength training; for example, do free weights one day and later in the week attend a power-pump class or a Pilates session.

Your First Step

Before you start using any type of equipment or strength-training system, you absolutely must learn how to do the exercises. This prevents injury. None of the systems are intuitively obvious to an uneducated beginner.

If you do a strength-training exercise incorrectly, the least that could happen is that you waste your time and energy. The worst … well … the worst ranges from minor to major injury. Somewhere in between is bulking up the wrong muscle.

Before you start, learn the correct moves:

◆ Read an instructional book or manual. Plenty are available at bookstores, online, and anywhere exercise equipment is sold.

◆ Take some classes. Learn the correct movements from a pro. Learn the proper plane of movement, the proper range of movement, the speed of movement, what muscle is being worked, and how many reps and sets are required to achieve your goal.

◆ Work with a certified personal trainer for one-on-one instruction. Most fitness centers offer personal training, or look in the Yellow Pages under fitness or personal trainers. Beware personal trainers who received their certifications in a weekend workshop.

◆ Take Pilates, Fitball, and other strength-training classes, either with a group or in a private one-on-one session.

◆ Work out along with exercise videos. They're inexpensive and at-home convenient. Collagevideo.com stocks hundreds of titles, and they sell small equipment, such as Fitballs, stretch tubing, body bars, and flex bands.

You'll have fun and get results even as you learn how to do strength training. You'll find there's always more to learn as you make progress.

THIN-couragement

Super slow, a new method of weight training, recommends doing very slow repetitions of each exercise, so that a person can't use any momentum in the movement. Momentum definitely makes a move easier. Find out whether this approach will work well for you by trying it. Overall, going slowly can be highly effective. You do fewer repetitions of each exercise, but take longer with each one.

Mindfulness

Unlike aerobic conditioning, where your mind can wander off while you huff and puff, strength training requires that you also engage your mind at the same time that you engage your muscles. Mentally focus on each movement as opposed to doing mindless reps, and your efforts will give you better results.

Concentration is key to your success. In fact, as you're doing the exercises, you may find yourself wishing that you could simply bliss out. But don't. Letting your mind wander can lead to injury.

Many people find strength training to be a form of meditation and relaxation because they can't dwell on their day-to-day concerns during a session.

Around the Middle

Losing inches from your waist and abdomen area is excellent for your physique and also great for your health. People who have high fat distribution around the midsection are more likely to develop chronic and life-threatening health conditions such as diabetes, heart disease, Alzheimer's, high blood pressure, and cancer.

You've already chosen to use glycemic index weight loss as a way to trim fat from your midsection. Use strength training as well.

Be sure that you do the following kinds of exercises and techniques to trim your entire midsection, known as your core:

◆ Good old-fashioned abdominal crunches are still the best basic exercise for your midsection. Make sure that you pull your navel into your spine as you do each crunch. Don't let your stomach pooch out as you do crunches because this will strengthen muscles that give you a potbelly.

◆ Whenever you do an exercise, think "navel to spine" and pull in your stomach.

◆ Do abdominal crunches, sit-ups, and roll-ups in which you work your waist and transverse abdominal muscles. One such exercise would be partial sit-ups done with your hands behind your head. As you sit up, touch your elbow to the opposite knee. These are tough, but very effective for toning the waist and abs.

◆ Do crunches and roll-ups on the Fitball. Ouch. The curve of the ball and the need for core stability as you do a crunch work the full range of your abdominal muscle group.

◆ Take a core-conditioning class to learn other exercises that strengthen and tone your core.

Many strength-training exercises target the abdominal muscles and the waist, so find your favorites and do those during your regular strength-training sessions.

A Daily Dose of Five Essential Exercises

Years ago, in 1939, a small book titled *Ancient Secret of the Fountain of Youth* was published. Written by Peter Keldor and published in the United States, it told the story of an aging colonel who went to Tibet and returned 10 years later, looking many years younger. The colonel attributed his youthful appearance to doing these five exercises every day. They're affectionately known as the Tibetans.

The story of the colonel in Tibet has never been verified, nor has anyone actually determined that the exercises originated in Tibet. But the power of the exercises is so amazing that a second book, *Ancient Secret of the Fountain of Youth Part 2* was published in 1998. It contains over 300 pages including the original book content. In the extra 200 pages, the authors attempt to explain why the Tibetan exercises work so well.

The Tibetans get your heart pumping, although not long enough for full cardio benefits. They strengthen your muscles and improve your flexibility. Even better, they give you a great lift, like you had a cup of coffee without the coffee.

The five Tibetans have been passed around quietly for years, and those of us who do them routinely would never stop. Why? Because they deliver. After you've done the five Tibetan exercises for about three months, you'll notice you no longer have a double chin. It vanishes. Women eventually discover that their midriffs are sort of slinkier, and men often have lost several belt sizes … even without losing weight.

THIN -couragement

On my 45th birthday, I, Lucy, received a copy of the *Ancient Secret of the Fountain of Youth* from my 19-year-old son. He gave me the book because, as he said, "Mom, you're getting old." Since that time, I have done the five simple Tibetan exercises faithfully every morning as I start my day. In just 5 to 10 minutes, I'm ready to take on whatever the day brings.

The reported benefits of the Tibetans are as follows:

- Double chin gone
- Midriff slimmer
- Upper arms firmer
- More energy
- Increased muscle tone
- Early morning wake-up lift

The following is what researchers say the five Tibetans do for the body:

- Stimulate the reticular activating system of the brain, making you more alert. Do before a college exam or important presentation.
- Balance the right and left hemispheres of the brain, which means you think more clearly.
- Balance the body's hormonal system.
- Strengthen bones because the exercises are weight bearing.
- Improve the body's immune system by stimulating all the organs and glands.
- Help the body detoxify by stimulating lymph movement.
- Build muscle strength.

- Reduce body-fat percentage.

- Boost metabolism.

- Align and strengthen the spine, making it more supple.

- Lighten menopausal symptoms.

- Lessen premenstrual symptoms.

- Help relieve the discomfort of arthritis and other aches and pains.

> **THIN-couragement**
>
> While Joe was on a three-month business trip to London, he did the Tibetan exercises twice a day, morning and late afternoon. He was careful to eat an amount of food the size of his fist three times a day. Plus he walked a lot. By the time he returned home to Australia, Joe had lost 4 inches around his waist. His wife didn't recognize him when he appeared at the front door. Joe was 56 years old.

Doing the Tibetans

We recommend that you do the Tibetans every morning when you wake up. They're easiest to do on an empty stomach. If the exercises seem too strenuous at first, refer to the book *Ancient Secret of the Fountain of Youth*, *Part 2*, published by Doubleday, for starter exercises so that you can slowly build up strength to do the full recommended set.

To begin, start with three or four repetitions of each exercise for the first week. Then increase the number of repetitions by a few every week until you reach the full 21 repetitions. Do the repetitions of each exercise before moving on to the next exercise. If you never work all the way up to 21 each, don't worry; they'll still deliver results.

The five Tibetan exercises can be performed anytime and virtually anywhere. It isn't necessary to do each exercise more than 21 times each to receive full benefit.

The Tibetans

Exercise 1: Standing with arms extended outward to your sides at shoulder height, spin your body toward your right hand. Go slowly at first and be sure to stop if you feel dizzy. Should you get dizzy, pick a spot on the wall and look at it until you feel clearheaded. Eventually, you will be able to spin quickly without getting dizzy. In the beginning, spin three complete rotations, eventually working up to 21.

Spinning seems like an odd exercise, and in a way it is. But it wakes your body up and seems to stimulate proper hormonal balance. There's a reason why children love to spin: it feels good and it's good for you.

Exercise 2: Lie flat on the floor, face up. Fully extend your arms along your sides and place the palms of your hands against the floor, keeping the fingers close together. If you want, place your hands under your hips to brace your movement. Then raise your head off the floor, tucking the chin against the chest. As you do this, lift your legs, knees straight, into a vertical position, perpendicular to the floor. If possible, let the legs extend back over the body toward the head, but do not bend your knees. Then slowly lower your head and legs, knees straight, to the floor to the beginning position. Breathe in deeply as you lift your legs and breathe out as you lower your legs again.

Exercise 1.

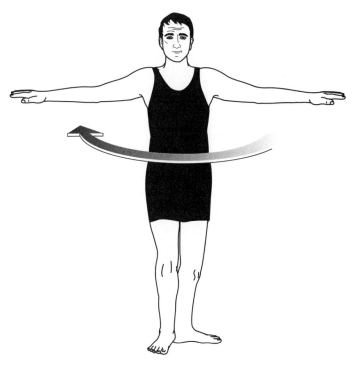

Exercise 2.

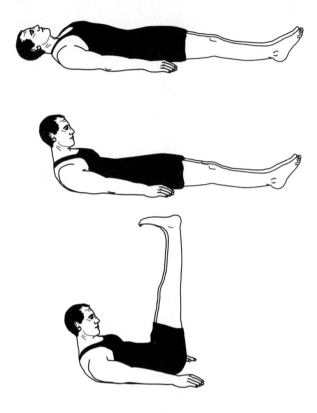

Exercise 3: Kneel on the floor with the torso of your body erect. Place your hands behind your back either in the middle back or lower back. Bend your neck and head forward, tucking the chin against the chest. Then gently move your head and neck backward slowly, arching your spine. As you arch, brace your hands against your body for support. Go backward until you are looking up at the ceiling and your neck feels fully stretched. Slowly return to the original position and start the second repetition. Breathe in deeply as you arch the spine and breathe out as you return to an erect position.

Exercise 4: Sit on the floor with your legs straight out in front of you and your feet about 12 inches apart. Sit up straight and place the palms of your hands on the floor alongside your buttocks, fingers pointed toward your toes. Tuck your chin forward against the chest. Then slowly drop your head backward as far as it will go. At the same time, raise your body so that the knees bend while the arms remain straight. The only body parts touching the floor are the palms of your hands and the soles of your feet.

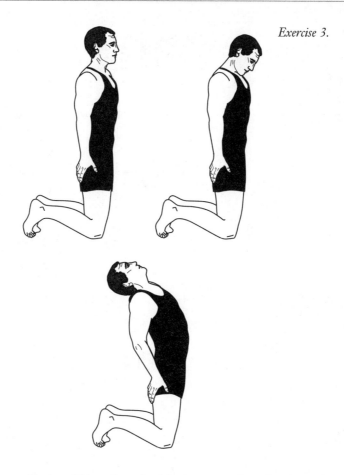

Exercise 3.

The trunk of your body will be aligned with the upper legs, horizontal to the floor. Your body will be in the shape of a bench. Then tense every muscle in the body. Finally, relax your muscles as you return to the original sitting position and rest before repeating the procedure. Breathe in as you raise up, hold your breath as you tense the muscles, and breathe out completely as you come down.

Exercise 5: When you perform the fifth exercise, your body is facing the floor with just your toes and hands on the floor. Make a tent shape out of your body, with your head tucked between your arms and your bottom up. Then move your torso toward the floor so that you are flexing the spine in reverse, and look up at the ceiling. Breathe in deeply as you raise your body and breathe out fully as you lower it. In yoga, these positions are called Downward Facing Dog and Upward Facing Dog.

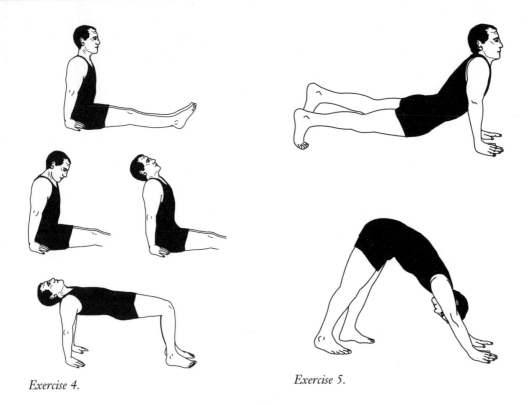

Exercise 4.

Exercise 5.

The five Tibetans are an exercise "extra" to boost your fitness progress. They're a great way to start the day, and they fit nicely with other parts of your exercise program. Clients rave about the results they get. You'll love the results, too.

The Least You Need to Know

◆ Strength training boosts your metabolism and reduces metabolic resistance to weight loss.

◆ Strength training quickly reduces body-fat percentage and increases muscle mass.

◆ Before you start a strength-training program, learn the correct way to do each exercise.

◆ Use strength training to keep your waist, midriff, and abdominal areas toned and trim.

◆ Do the five Tibetans every day upon waking; they feel good and do great things for you and your body.

Chapter 28

Stretching for Weight Loss

In This Chapter

- ◆ Stretching your way to weight loss
- ◆ Reducing cortisol levels and easing aches and pains
- ◆ Learning how to stretch
- ◆ Stretching to tone and flatten your tummy

Cats, dogs, and other animals do it. We're not so sure about the birds and the bees, but we know for certain that only some people do it. Which is too bad, because everyone can benefit from doing it regularly.

Yes, we're talking about stretching. Until recently, stretching was thought of as an exercise-program add-on. Exercise experts agreed that stretching was a good practice for staying limber and reducing injury, but fitness centers didn't offer stretching classes. At best, it was recommended that a person stretch for five minutes before or after aerobic exercise. How unfortunate.

Stretching is the third and final aspect of your complete exercise routine. In this chapter, you learn how stretching enhances your glycemic index weight-loss efforts and you learn the long and short of flexible-muscle maintenance.

Stretching Connection

It's not immediately obvious that there's a connection between stretching and weight loss. You don't burn more calories when you stretch. In fact, you hardly use any energy at all. Stretching has little to do with eating, except for the fact that it's difficult to eat when stretching. Your stretching time is time away from food, but that could hardly enhance your weight-loss efforts. So just how are glycemic index weight loss and stretching connected?

The Cortisol Connection

In previous chapters, we discussed that when your stress level rises, so does your body's level of the hormone insulin. This leads to insulin resistance and, ultimately, weight gain. So keeping your stress levels low also benefits weight loss.

Here's how stretching fits into this cortisol/insulin situation. When you're stressed, your muscles tighten. You've probably noticed that your shoulders seem to turn into rock solid knots as you work frantically on your keyboard to meet a deadline or spend screen time surfing the web or playing a video game.

You may also be familiar with tension headaches. A stressful situation prompts you to get tense, your muscles tighten, and before long you have a tension headache, a back-ache, or a leg cramp. We all carry stress in our muscles.

You must remove the stress from your muscles to release it. Stretching does just that. Many people have found that the secret to relieving headaches and backaches isn't found in the medicine cabinet or with a professional massage, but rather in taking five to ten minutes or more to stretch.

Stretching removes muscular tensions, lightens stress loads, and reduces cortisol levels, making it easier to lose weight.

Muscle Strain

Any time you use your muscles in new ways, you can experience a buildup of muscular tension and tightness. Activities that can cause muscular tension include strength training, sprains, aerobic exercise, anger, fear, anxiety, accidents, surgeries, illness, and even allergies. Even toting a heavy carry-on bag or briefcase through the airport can leave shoulders, arms, and even fingers tense, creating muscle aches and tightness.

The first reason this is a problem is that the tension makes your muscles hurt and the aches can last for days. The second reason is that the same aching muscles are the result of inflammation and increase your cortisol levels. How can you solve both problems? You guessed it—stretch out those muscles. Not only will you lower your cortisol levels, you may also find that the actual situation that caused the tension improves.

The bottom line here is this: muscle tension of any kind increases cortisol levels. Stretching releases muscle tension, lowers cortisol levels, and speeds up healing.

Stretching as Detox

When you stretch your muscles, you're helping to release toxins that are stored in fat and muscle. Stretching also helps move the lymph fluid that removes toxins through the body. Because toxin buildup can thwart weight loss, removing those toxins by stretching can further assist your glycemic index weight-loss efforts. See Chapter 25 for more information on how toxins are stored in fat.

Aches and Pains

If you've dealt with serious aches and pains in your life, such as chronic back pain, you know how easily pain and discomfort gets in the way of losing weight. Even if you eat correctly, the pain can be a barrier against getting to your ideal size. It makes exercise unappealing, because it can be painful to move.

Many doctors and physical therapists now use combination therapies to reduce pain. They continue to prescribe medicines and massage, but they also recommend stretching exercises to help reduce chronic pain and the stress caused by the pain, as well as to increase the range of movement. Again, the bottom line is this: less pain means less stress, which results in lowered cortisol levels, which lowers insulin levels, which promotes weight loss.

THIN -couragement

Joe was 45 when he began a stretching routine. He enjoyed racquetball and fencing, but found that he had trouble walking down steps the following mornings. His body was stiff and sore. His first five or ten stretching classes seemed brutal, as he was releasing athletic tensions and muscle bulk built up over the years. Within a couple of months, he noticed the stretching was easier and he was trading bulk and heft for a more graceful, yet strong body. His new muscle agility reduced his "morning-after racquetball" aches and pains.

Day-to-Day Stress

If your life is basically in balance, you're experiencing only normal, everyday stress. Still, stretching can assist you in regulating your cortisol levels and easing your way to weight loss. Use stretching to soothe your moods, refresh your body, and work out the kinks that result from normal daily activities and your exercise program.

THIN**-couragement**

Practically speaking, agility is important for regular living. Agility enables you to easily bend over, climb steps, and do basic everyday movements, such as tying your shoes and unloading the dishwasher. You need agility for all sorts of simple movements, not to mention being able to enjoy getting out on the dance floor and kicking up your heels.

Preventing Injuries

Traditionally, stretching has been recommended by exercise specialists as a way to reduce the likelihood of sports-related and exercise-related injuries. Flexible athletes can better withstand the bodily assaults they experience from contact sports and repetitive movements. In fact, many professional athletes—think football and basketball players—now participate in yoga and Pilates classes as a way to keep their muscles stretched, agile, and flexible.

Most likely, you aren't a professional athlete, but you can use stretching to receive the same benefits. Now that you're doing regular aerobic exercise and strength training, you need stretching to continue your fitness training comfortably for years to come.

Wrong Weigh

Don't think of stretching as too slow and tedious. The results are anything but. If you have hefty and strong thigh muscles that resist trimming, stretching will make them leaner. But it would take a while for stretching to break down the strong muscle fibers and elongate them. Go the distance with stretching—it brings wonderful rewards.

The Illusion of Slim

Having a longer and elongated body through stretching makes you appear slimmer as you lose weight. Your clothes will fit better and your posture will improve. Looking better and feeling better about the way you look motivates you to continue your glycemic index weight-loss efforts.

Getting Started

You are already a "natural" for stretching. You don't need to have lots of skill, but simply desire and some time. You don't need any equipment, but the following can be helpful:

- ◆ Clothing that is nonbinding and lets you move. You can wear a T-shirt and athletic-type shorts. You can also wear stretch clothing, such as a leotard and tights, or yoga pants and top.

- ◆ No shoes are required.

- ◆ A sticky mat that can be rolled up is useful, but not necessary.

Set aside time to stretch. Plan to stretch for 10 to 15 minutes at least every other day. Again, more is better. Add it onto the end of your regular exercise program, or set aside time in the evenings after work.

The most important rule in stretching, whether you're a beginner or more advanced, is this: *never overdo it.* Don't try to stretch farther than your muscles can comfortably release. When you stretch a muscle, your body sends you clear signals regarding how much is enough. It's painful to overdo it, and you could pull a muscle.

Exercise physiologists recommend warming up for two to five minutes before you begin stretching to prevent muscle pulls. The warm-up increases circulation and body heat, which makes your muscles stretch easier. Warm-up activities include walking, climbing stairs, and jogging.

Wrong Weigh

For travel, you don't need to pack along a heavy and bulky exercise mat. Instead, purchase a 5 foot roll of kitchen shelf liner that's sort of thick and rubbery. At your hotel, place a towel on the floor, top with the shelf liner and voilà, you're ready to move and stretch.

THIN-couragement

Even though stretching is easiest in loose-fitting clothing, don't let the wrong attire prevent you from stretching at your desk or on the floor of your office during a break. You may want to keep a yoga-type sticky mat in your office for stretch breaks.

For successful and effective stretching, follow this simple advice. Go slow to go fast. Take your time and pretty soon you, too, will be putting your hands on the floor when you bend over to touch your toes. All it takes is patience, tenacity, and perseverance. If your muscles hurt, then back off and only stretch as far as you are comfortable.

When you see a person who seems highly flexible, ask how long it took him or her to get to that level. Some people are simply born flexible, but most people need to acquire flexibility over time. If you've never stretched before in your life, expect to find it challenging to stretch and attain body flexibility. But don't give up. The results are a flexible body and mind.

Where and When to Stretch

You can stretch almost anywhere you have some space and relative privacy. Good locations and times for stretching include the following:

- At your desk. You'll be amazed at how many stretches you can do while seated in your office chair.

- On the floor of your office. Use a sticky mat or towel.

- Before and after aerobic exercise. Keeps your calves, hamstrings, and Achilles tendon flexible and supple.

- After strength training. Helps pull the buildup of lactic acid from your muscles that can cause soreness the next day. If you're still sore the next day, stretch again.

- While watching television. Get down on the floor and stretch during your favorite shows.

- While in the kitchen preparing meals. Usually the kitchen counter is just the right height for leg extension stretches (like ballerinas would do at the barre).

- At fitness classes, such as yoga and Pilates mat classes.

- After long periods spent sitting, as in car trips, airplane travel, seminars, or meetings.

Wrong Weigh

Be sure to hold each stretch when you reach your maximum stretch position. Don't bounce, but rather hold the position for 20 seconds to 2 minutes. As you do this, your muscles release and tensions melt away.

◆ First thing in the morning when you get out of bed or after your morning shower. Especially great if you're dealing with chronic aches and pains.

◆ When you get home from work as a way to decompress and relax.

◆ Before bed to relax before sleep.

Stretching is flexible, no pun intended. You can stretch virtually anywhere and relish the benefits wherever you happen to be.

Learning How to Stretch

Stretching is a very safe and comfortable activity, but even so, you need to learn which muscles to stretch and how. Use one or more of the following learning tools:

◆ An instructor, such as a yoga teacher, physical therapist, Pilates instructor, or fitness trainer.

◆ A book. One classic book that's been used for more than 25 years is *Stretching*, by Bob Anderson. Purchase at bookstores or online.

◆ Exercise videos and DVDs. These offer at-home learning. A good selection of offerings can be found at collagevideo.com.

◆ Take several basic stretching fitness classes. Unfortunately, you can't always rely on yoga classes to teach you the basics of stretching. Some are too exotic or unbalanced in their approach.

After you learn the basics of stretching your basic muscle groups, there is still more to learn. But you should first learn how to stretch your basic major muscle groups before moving on to advanced stretching.

THIN **-couragement**

If you're frustrated because you can't seem to lose weight and your muscles are strong and bulky, use this approach: cut back on your strength training and increase the time you spend stretching. The stretching will help elongate muscles and reduce bulk, thus enhancing your weight-loss momentum. Alternate aerobics and strength-training days, and stretch every day.

Stretching Methods

As you delve into stretching, you'll find several different methods and systems. Because stretching is as ancient as humankind, and because you have only a limited number of muscles that can be stretched, the systems are fundamentally the same. You can choose from any of the methods listed here:

◆ Yoga is an ancient system for stretching and well-being. Hatha yoga, the yoga of body movement, has many branches, such as Iyengar, Bikram, Astanga, and others. If you're just starting out, take a class that works with the basics. You can explore the other forms in depth later if you're so inclined. The yoga offered at most fitness centers is basic Hatha yoga.

◆ All-American stretching, as explained in the book *Stretching*, by Bob Anderson.

◆ Pilates is a recent exercise form that incorporates core strengthening with muscle toning and superb stretching. In one class you do both strength training and stretching. Pilates builds long, lean muscles and corrects any postural misalignments. You'll even stand up straighter.

◆ You can use equipment in your stretching that can intensify the stretch and enhance your workout. Such equipment includes flex bands, stretch tubing, and Fitballs.

All three aspects of exercise—aerobic conditioning, strength training, and stretching—work synergistically to give you the shape, stamina, and health you desire.

Streamline Your Tummy and Waist

Streamlining your tummy may seem like fantasy to you. By now you know that sit-ups and crunches don't make your tummy flat no matter how many you do. In fact, the more you do, the bigger your midsection seems.

There is a way to flatten, slim, and streamline, and it works perfectly with glycemic index weight loss. By eating low glycemic, you're not eating the foods that cause midsection bulge. By keeping your stress levels lower, you're not adding worry weight to your waist.

You can streamline your middle by a combination of stretching and other exercises and activities.

Stretching Your Midsection

As we age, our spines get shorter and our midsection gets wider. Part of this is cause and effect. A tall glass jar filled with water can contain as much water as a shorter wide jar. By elongating your spine through stretching and other techniques, your midsection gets smaller.

Stretching is the step beyond sit-ups and crunches for minimizing your midsection. You'll love the results. Here are the stretches to use:

◆ Do reverse abdominal stretching after your crunches and sit-ups. Roll back over a large Fitball so that you're facing up, with your hands touching the floor behind you and your feet or toes on the floor in front. This stretches your abs as well as the psoas muscles that run from the side of your abdomen down the front side of your leg. Roll slowly and feel each vertebra lengthen.

◆ Lie over a Fitball facing the floor with your stomach on the ball. Very slowly, roll on the ball—pausing as each vertebra receives an elongating stretch.

◆ Stretch your body laterally—that is, to the side. Target the muscles that run from the sides of your legs up through the sides of your torso. You can do this on the Fitball by reclining on your side. Or stand and stretch slowly to one side and then to the other side. Sit on the floor with legs apart and bend over laterally to touch the toes on one foot. Hold. And then stretch to the other foot. Often, we've found that stretching- and yoga-class instructors forget to teach these important slimming lateral stretches.

> **THIN-couragement**
>
> To have a tight and flat abdominal area, you need to stretch your abdominal area muscles as well as strengthen them with crunches, sit-ups, and other core training exercises. Don't omit the stretching. It can reduce bulky muscles and smooth out the way your gut looks.

Experiment with stretches. When you find ones that target your specific needs, use them often to regain your youthful figure.

Flatten Your Tummy

We searched for additional techniques as we've encountered the inevitable broadening midsection. The following suggestions flatten the tummy and elongate the spine. We know from experience that they work.

Use an Inversion Machine. You'll hang upside down from your ankles. Everything stretches. The machine was developed to help relieve back pain due to compressed spinal disks. You'll use it to elongate your entire body, spine included. Hang a couple times a week for 5 to 10 minutes. The experience feels oddly good. Purchase at back stores and online.

Do Body Rolling. Especially up your tummy, along your upper hips, and your spine. The whole process is superbly relaxing. You can do body rolling every day or several times a week to start. Plan on maintaining your flat tummy with body-rolling sessions once or twice a month. Purchase Body Rolling balls and instructions online. The book *The Ultimate Body Rolling Workout,* by Yamuna Zake, explains everything.

Do the Yoga Abdominal Muscle Lock. When standing up, blow out all the air in your lungs. Then quickly pull in your abdominal muscles very tightly and suck in your gut. Hold your breath without inhaling for a count of ten. Then inhale, relaxing your tummy muscles. Do three times once a day. This sounds odd, is odd, and really works fast. You can also do the Abs Lock when stopped at traffic lights or in the shower.

The Least You Need to Know

◆ Add a stretching routine to your exercise program to enhance your ability to lose weight.

◆ Stretching makes you look slimmer and can help decrease the size of bulky muscles.

◆ Stretching helps reduce cortisol levels, detoxify the body, and soothe moods.

◆ Do at least two 15-minute stretching sessions a week, but more is better.

◆ Elongate and flatten your tummy with stretching exercises.

Glossary

aerobic exercise   Exercise that you do for a sustained amount of time, for at least 15 minutes, that moves your major muscles and makes you huff and puff and break into a sweat. Running, jogging, swimming, and bicycling are popular forms. But vigorous hiking, racquetball, tennis, or dancing are also considered aerobic exercise, as are aerobic conditioning classes. Golf, bowling, and billiards aren't.

alkaline ash effect   The result of urine turning more alkaline. When the body is slightly alkaline, it's easier for it to maintain the proper bacteria-yeast balance level so that a person can reduce or eliminate urinary tract infections as well as yeast infections.

amino acids   The chemical units that make up protein. The nine essential amino acids required for health must be ingested. Foods that contain all nine are designated complete protein foods. Foods that do not contain all nine essential amino acids are called incomplete proteins.

basal metabolic rate   The rate at which a person's body uses energy in a resting state, such as sitting still. The body really does "burn" through food, actually producing heat and providing energy to your organs and muscles.

blood sugar level   Your blood sugar level is considered healthy when the fasting level is between 80 and 120. This can be measured at a doctor's office.

body burden   The amount of toxins an individual has in the body at any point in time.

body fat percentage   A measurement of a person's body fat. The total amount of body fat, muscle mass, and water a person has equals 100 percent. Body fat percentage can be measured at a health center, a doctor's office, or a fitness club.

brain fog   A popular phrase to describe the state of being mentally fuzzy or unable to think coherently.

celiac disease   A chronic digestive disorder caused by an inherited intolerance to gluten, a component of wheat, rye, oats, and barley. May cause malabsorption of nutrients and food allergies. May be quite serious if left untreated. The first step in treatment is to avoid eating foods containing gluten.

cold expeller pressed   A method for extracting vegetable oils that uses a cold method which best preserves nutrients and flavor. Hot expeller presses heat the oils and can destroy nutrients and alter taste.

complete proteins   Foods that contain all nine essential amino acids. Proteins from meat, fish, fowl, shellfish, and dairy are complete proteins. Cheeses offer more protein per ounce than milk and yogurt.

cortisol   A stress hormone secreted by the adrenal glands that stimulates the release of glycogen stores in the liver and in the muscles. Glycogen is the body's storage form of carbohydrate that breaks down into blood glucose in times of need. The extra blood glucose produced by cortisol increases stamina, endurance, and mental acuity during times of stress. Cortisol levels are high when a person's short- or long-term stress is high. Elevated cortisol levels often lead to such chronic conditions as weight gain, diabetes, heart disease, cancer, and high blood pressure.

essential fatty acids (EFAs)   Polyunsaturated fats that are essential for your health. They can be obtained only by ingesting them, thus the government designation of "essential." The two main essential fatty acids are alpha-linolenic acid (an omega-3 fatty acid), and linoleic acid (an omega-6 fatty acid).

fruit ogliosaccharide (FOS)   A probiotic nutritional supplement that selectively nourishes the friendly bacteria in the intestines. It increases the number of good bacteria in your gut. FOSs are definitely good for you.

glycemic load   Measures the total impact of an amount of food on blood sugar levels. To calculate the load, multiply the number of grams of carbohydrate in a food by its glycemic index.

glyconutrients   Sugars that naturally occur in plants. Some, such as galactose (a milk sugar) and glucose, taste sweet. The others are not sweet. All are needed by the body for important metabolic processes.

HDL   High-density lipoproteins are known as the "good cholesterol." Low HDL cholesterol levels (less than 40 mg/dL) increase the risk for heart disease. HDL is considered protective to the body's cardiovascular health, in contrast to "bad" LDL cholesterol.

high-glycemic foods   Carbohydrates that trigger a quick rise in blood sugar levels. These are such foods as bread, cookies, sodas, white potatoes, some packaged break-fast cereals, and highly refined grains. Low-glycemic foods are foods such as green vegetables, many fruits, legumes, and nuts that cause a slight and safe rise in blood sugar levels. Medium-glycemic foods include table sugar, some dried fruits, and some whole-grain crackers and breads that cause a moderate rise. In the induction phase of a low-carb weight-loss program, you eat only low-glycemic carbohydrates. See Appendix B for a listing of the glycemic index of many foods.

incomplete proteins   Foods that don't contain all nine essential amino acids. These foods are vegetables or vegetable based, such as soybeans, nuts, legumes, and grains.

induction phase   A standard part of low-carb as opposed to low-glycemic weight-loss programs. In the two-week induction phase, a person eats strictly limited amounts of carbohydrates, most of which are "free vegetables." Induction phase eating is out of balance and not necessary for weight loss.

insulin resistance   A condition that occurs when the body's cells no longer readily uptake glucose for energy from insulin. The cells are then, in a sense, unable to respond to insulin.

insulin sensitivity   A term that indicates the body's cells respond to insulin correctly. This is the opposite of insulin resistance, in which the body's cells don't respond adequately to insulin and thus don't absorb nutrients, such as blood sugar, efficiently.

ketone bodies   The by-products of fat metabolism. They're made by the liver and are a normal part of metabolism. On a low-carb weight-loss program, the liver makes more ketone bodies than at other times. The amount of ketone bodies produced is indicated on ketone urine strips.

ketosis   The process of making ketone bodies from lipolysis. The ketone bodies are then used for energy. As your body uses its fat for energy, you lose weight.

LDL   High levels of LDL (low-density lipoprotein) cholesterol can signal medical problems like cardiovascular disease, it is sometimes called "bad cholesterol" (as opposed to HDL, the "good cholesterol").

lipolysis   The breakdown of fat, known as triglycerides, into free fatty acids and glycerol. These fatty acids are then used as energy to fuel the body. Insulin inhibits lipolysis and favors fat storage.

metabolic resistance   A condition in which a person's basal metabolic rate is so low that the person has a difficult time losing weight.

metabolism   The rate at which your body burns fuel. A high metabolism makes it easier for a person to lose weight and keep it off. Having a slow metabolism makes it harder to lose weight. You can increase your metabolism through exercise and by eating the low-glycemic way.

monounsaturated fats   Dietary fats that are highly beneficial to your health and to losing weight. They are typically liquid at room temperature but solidify when refrigerated.

mystery ingredients   Food package ingredients that you can't pronounce are ingredients that you can't easily purchase by themselves at the grocery store (for example, maltodextrins), or are preservatives and artificial colorings. Avoid purchasing products with more than two or three mystery ingredients, if any.

net carbs   The total amount of carbohydrates in a food serving minus dietary fiber and any added sugar alcohols. Net carbs give a good indication of how a food will affect blood sugar levels. Dietary fiber doesn't raise blood sugar levels. Even though sugar alcohol is not a true carbohydrate or a true alcohol, it will raise a person's blood glucose level to a small degree. If you are diabetic, count one half of the sugar alcohol grams as part of your total carbohydrate intake.

nutrient dense   Foods that naturally contain high concentrations of essential nutrients, such as complete protein, essential fatty acids, vitamins, minerals, or antioxidants.

phytonutrients   The nutrients found in plants and plant products, such as vegetables, fruits, nuts, and seeds. Phytonutrients include vitamins, minerals, antioxidants, and glyconutrients.

Pilates   An exercise form that originated with Joseph Pilates in the 1940s. It focuses on strengthening the core muscles, which are in the abdominal area. The exercises combine strength training and stretching. The result is long, lean, flexible, and strong muscles, plus great posture.

polyunsaturated fats   Dietary fats whose molecules are not "saturated" with hydrogen atoms due to the presence of two or more double carbon bonds. Polyunsaturated fats are liquid at room temperature and remain liquid when refrigerated or frozen.

saccharides   The scientific term for sugars. The term includes all sugars, including the sugars we intentionally eat, such as sucrose, fructose, and lactose (the sugar in milk). Saccharides also include other lesser-known sugars present in foods that don't raise blood sugar levels and that are considered non-nutritive because they don't contain calories.

saturated fat   A molecular structure that is saturated with hydrogen atoms. Saturated fats are solid at room temperature. Butter and lard are saturated fats.

serotonin   A brain neurotransmitter responsible for relaxation and uplifted moods.

starvation metabolism   A general slow-down of body metabolism often caused by not eating enough calories as in starvation diets. May cause an increase in body fat and the inability to lose weight.

stevia with FOS   A natural low-calorie and low-carbohydrate sweetener. In its pure state, it's 10 times sweeter than sugar with virtually no carbohydrates or calories. Stevia is an herb that originated in South America, and FOSs are fruit ogliosaccharides that nourish the friendly bacteria in the intestines that support gastrointestinal health. Just ¼ teaspoon is equivalent in sweetness to 1 teaspoon of sugar.

toxins   Chemical substances that harm or irritate the body. A person can get toxins into the body through breathing, consuming them when eating, drinking, or taking medications, and through skin contact.

trace minerals   Minerals required by the body in extremely small amounts. They aid metabolic processes.

trans-fatty acids   Fats that are manmade by converting unsaturated vegetable oils into partially hydrogenated vegetable oils through heating, at which time hydrogen atoms become attached to the oils. Partially hydrogenated fats are solids at room temperature and are more chemically stable, meaning that they have a longer shelf life than an unsaturated vegetable oil. Trans-fatty acids have been shown to directly cause clogged arteries and heart disease. They are found in many commercially available baked goods and other processed foods. The FDA requires that all food labels list the amount of trans fats per serving.

trigger food   A food that can lead you to overeating, or even to binge eating. Some common trigger foods are candy, chips, popcorn, donuts, and ice cream. If you have a trigger food and find it impossible to eat only a small amount, it's best not to eat it at all.

Food Listings for Carbohydrates, Glycemic Index, and Glycemic Load

This list includes only information on foods that contain carbohydrates. Animal proteins, such as meats, seafood, and poultry, don't contain carbohydrates, so their glycemic index and glycemic load are both zero. The same is true for butter and vegetable oils.

High glycemic—over 70

Medium glycemic—56–69

Low glycemic—55 and under

Foods	Glycemic Index Value	Amount	Carbs in Grams	Fiber in Grams	Net Carbs	Glycemic Load
Almond flour	0	1 cup	21	11	10	0
Almonds	0	1 cup	28	15	13	0
Apple juice	40	1 cup	29	0	29	12
Apples	38	1 medium	22	5	17	6
Apples, dried	29	9 rings	37	5	32	9
Applesauce, unsweetened	40	½ cup	13	3	10	6
Apricots	57	3 medium	10	1	9	5
Apricots, dried	30	¼ cup	29	2	27	8
Artichokes	0	½ cup	6	4	2	0
Avocado, California	0	1 medium	12	9	3	0
Bagel	72	1 small	30	0	30	22
Baked beans	50	½ cup	27	7	11	20
Banana	52	1 medium	29	4	25	12
Barley, pearl, uncooked	25	¼ cup	37	6	31	11
Barley, rolled, cooked	66	½ cup	15	2	13	9
Basmati brown rice, cooked	58	½ cup	18	2	16	8
Beets, canned	64	½ cup	6	1	5	3
Black beans, boiled	30	½ cup	20	8	12	4
Black-eyed peas, canned	42	½ cup	16	4	12	5
Bouillon, chicken or beef	0	½ cup	2	0	0	0
Bran, whole wheat	0	2 TB.	5	3	2	0
Brazil nut	0	6 large	4	2	0	0
Bread, flat, whole-grain rye	48	1 oz.	15	2	13	6
Bread, 100% whole grain	51	1 slice	13	2	11	7
Bread, sourdough wheat	54	1 slice	15	1	14	7
Bread, sourdough rye	48	1 slice	15	1	14	6

Foods	Glycemic Index Value	Amount	Carbs in Grams	Fiber in Grams	Net Carbs	Glycemic Load
Bread, white	80	1 slice	15	1	14	11
Bread, whole wheat	77	1 slice	15	1	14	9
Broccoli, raw, chopped	0	½ cup	2	1	1	0
Brown sugar	59	1 oz.	28	0	28	17
Cabbage, raw, shredded	0	½ cup	2	1	1	0
Cantaloupe, cubed	65	1 cup	13	2	11	6
Capers	0	1 TB.	1	0	1	0
Carrots, raw, shredded	47	½ cup	6	2	4	3
Cashews	22	½ cup	8	3	5	3
Cassava	46	½ cup	15	1	14	6
Cauliflower, 1-inch pieces	0	½ cup	3	2	1	0
Celery, diced	0	½ cup	2	1	1	0
Cereals						
All-Bran or Fiber One	30	½ cup	24	14	10	3
Bran Chex	58	½ cup	23	4	19	11
Bran flakes	74	½ cup	22	4	18	13
Cheerios	74	½ cup	11	1	10	7
Cornflakes	92	½ cup	12	1	11	10
Cream of Wheat, cooked	74	½ cup	15	1	14	10
Grape Nuts	75	½ cup	31	2	29	22
Oatmeal, instant, cooked	66	½ cup	15	1	14	9
Oatmeal, thick-cut, cooked	53	½ cup	15	2	13	7
Rice Krispies	82	½ cup	11	1	10	8
Shredded Wheat	75	½ cup	15	2	13	10
Cheese, cheddar and Parmesan	0	1 oz.	0	0	0	0
Cherries, sweet with pits	22	½ cup	12	2	10	2
Chèvre cheese	0	1 oz.	1	0	1	0
Chickpeas, canned	42	½ cup	18	7	11	7

continues

continued

Foods	Glycemic Index Value	Amount	Carbs in Grams	Fiber in Grams	Net Carbs	Glycemic Load
Chocolate milk, low-fat	34	1 cup	26	0	26	9
Cocoa powder	55	1 TB.	3	1	2	1
Corn, sweet, boiled	60	½ cup	23	5	18	11
Cornmeal	68	¼ cup	25	3	22	5
Couscous	65	¼ cup	13	2	11	7
Crackers						
Soda crackers	74	6 squares	15	0	15	11
Wheat Thins	67	1 oz.	20	1	19	13
Cream, heavy	0	½ cup	3	0	3	0
Cucumber, sliced	0	½ cup	1.4	1	0	0
Dates	50	¼ cup	32	3	29	15
Donut, cake	76	1 small	23	0	23	17
Eggs, large	0	1 large	0.6	0	0.6	0
Fennel, sliced	0	1 cup	6	2	4	0
Figs, dried	61	3 figs	31	5	26	15
Garlic	0	1 clove	1	0.1	1	0
Grapefruit	25	½ medium	16	6	10	3
Grapefruit juice	48	1 cup	20	0	20	9
Grapes, green	46	¾ cup	19	1	18	8
Green beans, cooked	0	½ cup	5	2	3	0
Green onions	0	¼ cup	2	1	1	0
Green peas, frozen	48	2/3 cup	12	4	8	6
Hazelnuts, diced	0	1 cup	18	7	11	0
Honey, varies widely	55-78	1 TB.	18	0	18	10–20
Ice cream, low fat, vanilla	50	½ cup	9	0	9	5
Jicama	0	½ cup	5	3	2	0
Kidney beans, boiled	46	½ cup	20	7	14	6
Kiwi fruit	58	1 medium	11	3	9	5
Leafy vegetables, raw	0	1 cup	2	1	1	0
Lentils, cooked	29	½ cup	20	8	12	3

Foods	Glycemic Index Value	Amount	Carbs in Grams	Fiber in Grams	Net Carbs	Glycemic Load
Lima beans, frozen	32	½ cup	22	5	17	7
Macadamia nuts	0	¼ cup	5	3	2	0
Mango, sliced	51	½ cup	18	3	15	8
Milk, 2%	32	1 cup	13	0	13	4
Millet, cooked	71	2/3 cup	38	2	36	25
Muesli, no sugar added	54	1 oz.	18	2	16	9
Navy beans, cooked	38	½ cup	36	5	31	12
Oat bran	55	2 TB.	10	5	5	3
Oatmeal, slow cooking, cooked	42	½ cup	13	2	11	5
Orange, sections	42	½ cup	13	2	11	3
Orange juice	53	1 cup	18	0	18	9
Papaya, sliced	56	½ cup	11	3	8	5
Parsnips (cooked)	97	½ cup	13	1	12	12
Pasta						
Spaghetti (cooked 15 minutes)	64	½ cup	16	1	15	10
Spaghetti (cooked 5 minutes)	38	½ cup	16	1	15	6
Spirali pasta (cooked 6 minutes)	43	½ cup	16	1	15	6
Whole-wheat spaghetti (cooked 5 minutes)	32	½ cup	16	2	14	5
Peach, sliced	42	1 cup	14	3	11	5
Peanuts, roasted	14	¼ cup	7	2	5	1
Pear	38	1 medium	25	4	21	4
Peas, frozen	48	½ cup	12	4	8	4
Pecan flour	0	1 cup	15	15	0	0
Pecans, halves	0	¼ cup	5	5	0	0
Pepper, red or green bell, diced	0	¾ cup	4	2	2	0
Pineapple, diced	66	½ cup	19	2	17	8

continues

continued

Foods	Glycemic Index Value	Amount	Carbs in Grams	Fiber in Grams	Net Carbs	Glycemic Load
Pine nuts or pinion nuts	0	¼ cup	5	2	3	0
Pinto beans, canned	45	½ cup	18	6	12	7
Plums, sliced	39	½ cup	11	1	10	5
Popcorn, microwaved	72	1½ cups	14	3	11	8
Potato, white, baked in skin	85	4¾×2½ inches	35	5	30	26
Potato chips	57	2 oz.	18	0	18	10
Pretzels	83	1 oz.	20	0	20	16
Prunes, pitted	29	6	34	4	30	9
Pumpkin, cooked	75	1 cup	15	3	12	9
Raisins	64	¼ cup	31	2	29	14
Rice, brown, cooked	50	¼ cup	37	3	35	16
Rice cakes	82	3 cakes	21	0	21	17
Rutabaga, cooked	72	½ cup	12	2	10	7
Salami	0	1 oz.	0	0	0	0
Soybeans, canned	14	1 cup	19	8	11	2
Split peas, cooked	32	¼ cup	27	11	16	2
Strawberries	40	½ cup	6	1	5	1
Sucrose, granulated table sugar	68	1 TB.	10	0	10	7
Sweet potato, mashed	44	½ cup	24	3	21	11
Taco shells, baked	68	2 small	32	2	30	20
Tapioca, cooked with milk	81	¾ cup	19	1	18	14
Tomato, chopped	28	1 cup	8	2	6	2
Tortilla chips, plain, salted	63	1 oz.	15	1	14	8
Walnuts, halves	0	¼ cup	3	3	0	0
Wild rice, uncooked	57	¼ cup	34	3	31	18
Yams, cooked, cubed	37	½ cup	39	3	36	13

Glycemic Index Diet Review

Today you can search on the Internet with the keywords "glycemic index" and pull up almost 1,500,000 sites or references. Yes, talk about the glycemic index is everywhere. Why? It works as no other weight loss or health program can.

The glycemic index approach to weight loss is shaking up traditional calorie- and fat gram–counting diet companies. They've added the glycemic index into their product mix.

With a wide variety of resources on the glycemic index for you to choose from, we've culled through the websites and bookstores and come up with our favorites. The books reviewed in this appendix could be valuable additions to your resources library.

The Glucose Revolution

The New Glucose Revolution: The Authoritative Guide to the Glycemic Index—the Dietary Solution for Lifelong Health

The New Glucose Revolution was the first book to popularize eating low-glycemic foods. It was first published in 1999 and is now in its third revision. The authors—Jennie Brand-Miller, Ph.D.; Thomas M. S. Wolever, M.D., Ph.D.; Kaye Foster-Powell, M. Nutr. & Diet; and Stephen Colagiuri, M.D.—are well versed in the science of carbohydrates and their effects on the body's insulin levels and blood glucose levels. They discuss the need for eating mostly low-glycemic carbohydrates and explain how high-glycemic carbohydrates aren't good for your health or waistline.

But, they explain, neither is eating too many low-glycemic carbohydrates. Their point is that the glycemic index of a particular carbohydrate reveals only half the equation. The other half is the glycemic load, which, as you know, mathematically takes into account the glycemic index of a food *and* the quantity eaten.

The authors recommend eating about 250 grams of carbs a day. They suggest that eating low-glycemic carbs promotes health, but suggest it's fine to eat medium- and even high-glycemic carbs—provided that an average person who's not on a weight-loss program eats a glycemic load of between 138 and 163 for the day.

What the Program Misses. The authors promote eating low- and medium-glycemic starches, even for people who want to lose weight, but don't discuss the prevalence of food allergies to wheat and other starches that can promote weight gain. For a dieter, they recommend four servings of breads, pasta, cereal, rice, or noodles per day. This is too much starch for many overweight people and certainly too much for people who are metabolically resistant to weight loss.

How It Hits the Mark. We sincerely thank the authors for their research on the glycemic index. Without their efforts and courage, we might never have been able to understand the biology of insulin resistance and the effects that carbohydrates have on weight gain and weight management.

The book was not written as a book on weight loss, but rather as a guide to healthy eating. The back of the book contains an extensive list of many carbohydrate foods, giving their glycemic index along with their glycemic load. The list includes many brand-name foods, including cereals and baked goods.

The New Glucose Revolution Shopper's Guide to GI Values 2008: The Authoritative Source of Glycemic Index Values for More Than 1000 Foods

Use this shopping guide by the authors of *The New Glucose Revolution*—Dr. Jennie Brand-Miller and Kaye Foster-Powell. It lists the glycemic index value for many farm-sourced and factory-sourced foods.

In addition you'll find nutritional information on serving size, calories, fat, saturated fat, carbohydrate, fiber, and sodium per serving for each food listed.

We applaud that the authors offer advice on how to eat low glycemic when on a gluten-free diet. Take along with you to the grocery store.

The Glycemic Index Diet

The GI Diet

The GI Diet was originally published in Canada, where it's been highly successful. The book's popularity has since spread to the United States. The author, Rick Gallop, offers a simple plan of low-glycemic eating combined with good fats and lean meats.

His latest book, *The GI Diet Express: for Busy People*, shows you how to incorporate glycemic index eating into a busy and hectic life. It includes shopping tips, recipes, and solid advice.

You won't find yourself counting or calculating in this plan; instead, you eat foods based on whether they're listed in the red, yellow, or green lists. Red foods are foods you should avoid or eat very infrequently. Yellow foods are marginally acceptable, but you won't eat much of them. By contrast, green foods are a "go." Eat them in moderate amounts and you'll lose weight and feel better.

You'll do plenty of healthful exercise by following the exercise guidelines and tracking your progress with the exercise diary forms. Plus, resistance training is included, which is great for everyone but is especially advantageous for a person who's metabolically resistant to weight loss.

What the Program Misses. *The GI Diet* offers simplified solutions that don't address topics such as stress hormones, body burden, and emotional eating. Still, even without these, anyone can follow the book's color-coded approach.

More significantly, the book doesn't address glycemic load at all, but instead gives you recommended serving sizes. If you use this program, be sure to carefully follow the program so that you don't overeat or eat too high a glycemic load.

The diet recommends limiting fats more than you need to. It's beneficial to weight loss to eat whole eggs in moderate amounts, but the diet puts whole eggs in the red zone. It also supports the use of artificial sweeteners that are known to stimulate appetite and lead to metabolic syndrome and whose safety is highly controversial.

How It Hits the Mark. If you want a very simple low-glycemic weight-loss program, this one can work well. The program is nutritionally sound, but extreme in strictly limiting fat. In fact, you'll lose weight on this program even if you ease up on the fat restrictions. Although it's true that eating too much overall fat can cause insulin resistance, what works best for weight control and decreasing insulin resistance is to eat about 20 percent to 35 percent of total calories from fat.

Eating too little fat—below 20% can decrease your ability to eat enough essential fatty acids for health and weight loss.

The Zone and Paleo Diets

The Zone

Now that *The Zone* is over 10 years old, it is considered to be a classic book on low-carb and low-glycemic eating. Barry Sears, the author, suggests that an ideally balanced diet is 30 percent protein, 30 percent fat, and 40 percent carbs, which can work for many people.

The Zone advocates eating lean meats, good fats, and low-glycemic carbohydrates. You'll be eating plenty of vegetables and fruits, so you're certain to eat at least 5, and more like 10, servings a day.

When *The Zone* was originally published, the concept that high-glycemic carbohydrates cause insulin resistance was new information. So was the distinction between good and bad fats.

The Zone is a good weight-loss program and can assist you in eating based on the glycemic index.

The Paleo Diet

Loren Cordaine used the point of view of evolutionary biology in developing his groundbreaking eating program. The premise is this: human DNA today is virtually identical to that of cavemen and cavewomen. The foods they ate for more than seven million years are the same foods that our bodies are still best adapted to digest and assimilate. And surprise, those foods are definitely low glycemic. All around, *The Paleo Diet* is a winner.

Cordaine's major premise is that our bodies are not as well suited to digest and assimilate foods that have only recently been introduced into the human diet. Makes sense so far. Now here's what's so surprising.

It's only been during the past 10,000 years that humans have eaten grains and dairy foods. That may seem like a long time, but 10,000 years is just a tick-tock of the clock compared to the previous seven million years of human evolution. Cordaine points out that many people have allergic reactions or food sensitivities to grains and dairy. But that's not all. Coffee, tea, refined sugar, enriched flour, artificial sweeteners, and chemical preservatives are even newer in the human diet and we are less suited to consume them, too.

By eating a Paleo Diet, Cordaine claims people can lose weight easily, maintain the weight loss, and stay healthier.

Caveperson foods are meats, fish, poultry, eggs, vegetables and fruits, nuts and seeds, and some honey. According to Cordaine, these foods contain all the nutrition anyone needed in the past or needs now. This only makes sense. If our ancient ancestors weren't able to obtain necessary nutrients from their foods, the human race would have died out millions of years ago.

Cordaine recommends that you avoid eating modern foods, such as foods made from grains including cereals, muffins, cookies, pancakes, and such. He also recommends that you avoid eating dairy products.

Cordaine doesn't make the distinction between farm-sourced foods and factory-sourced foods, but his recommended foods are primarily farm-sourced.

On the Paleo Diet, you won't eat starches, dairy, refined sugars, or sodas. This means your carbohydrate intake will limit itself naturally to low-glycemic foods. If you take away the carbohydrates introduced into the human diet within the past 10,000 years, the only ones left are vegetables, fruits, nuts, seeds, and honey. They're basically all low glycemic. (The glycemic index for honey ranges widely, but some honeys are low glycemic.)

The program isn't strict, but it certainly can be called restrictive. And yes, you can cheat. Some. For instance, the author admits to a fondness for wine, and we're sure you could figure out how to eat some chocolate and still be 90 percent faithful to eating like your "inner caveperson." The book advocates getting plenty of hearty exercise just as our ancient ancestors did daily.

What the Program Misses. The Paleo Diet doesn't miss. The science is solid and the program quite simply works. Cordaine covers glycemic index, glycemic load, and the need to avoid overeating.

It's unrealistic to think that many people could easily give up the all-enticing nuances of modern-day factory-sourced foods and revert to primitive eating, but we find the information helpful in understanding our genetics and the basics of healthy eating.

How It Hits the Mark. The program is so simple that anyone can understand it. There's no weighing and no measuring. You don't even need to count. You might find it tricky to eat a meal at the baseball stadium, but then, you would also find it tricky to eat at the baseball stadium based on any glycemic index weight-loss program.

If you are plagued with allergies, candida, high blood pressure, heart disease, diabetes, fatigue, mood disorders, autoimmune diseases, or other chronic health problems, give the Paleo Diet a try and eat as a caveperson would for a month or two. You might be amazed at your results and with your weight loss. The recommended foods don't trigger cortisol release, so they can help lighten your stress load and emotional eating patterns.

The Detox Diet

The Fast Track Detox Diet: Boost metabolism, get rid of fattening toxins, jump-start weight loss and keep the pounds off for good

The author, Ann Louise Gittleman, PhD., C.N.S., speaks to the heart of the weight-loss conundrum. Women want to look younger and be healthier fast. Her methods offer everything you need—including up-to-date science—to detoxify your body and feel great while reaching your ideal size. Gittleman is concerned about a person's total health, including emotional well-being. She presents a totally comprehensive plan that includes all aspects of lifestyle as it relates to weight gain and weight loss. You'll find information about ways to eat low glycemic while enjoying good fats and lean meats. Plus, it includes a specific exercise program, ways to combat stress-related weight gain, and a method to detoxify your body so that your body can flush out the fat from your hips, waist, and thighs.

In Gittleman's book, you'll find biological and nutritional explanations of all the elements of the program. You'll learn how the liver removes toxins from the body and how it functions to release stored fat. The explanations are clear and useful.

The program is integrated into every area of your life, from what you do upon rising in the morning to going to sleep at night. In between those times, you do detoxifying physical exercises, drink cranberry and long-life cocktails, and journal.

The Fast Track Detox appeals specifically to middle-aged women who are wrestling with weight gain due to hormonal imbalances. The author understands this frustration and many women in their 40s, 50s, and 60s have experienced success with this program.

What the Program Misses. We can't think of a thing wrong from a health point of view. However, compliance with this eating plan requires high commitment and mindfulness.

How It Hits the Mark. If you want a totally comprehensive low-glycemic lifestyle program, this one's for you. The program is very specific and rigorous, so be prepared to eat the recommended foods and to follow the program carefully. Doing the program comprehensively takes time and planning, and the ability to afford organic produce and other specialty food products.

This program works well if you're metabolically resistant to weight loss or have midlife hormonal concerns. If you know that you've been exposed to heavy doses of environmental toxins that could be affecting your health or your life, give the Fast Track Detox Plan a try. Also consider using this program if you have weight gain specifically around your midsection.

The Atkins Diet

Dr. Atkins's New Diet Revolution

And what a revolution he created! Dr. Robert Atkins was the first to advise us to stop counting calories and, instead, to count carbohydrates. That was in the early 1970s. Needless to say, the medical and dietetic communities didn't warmly embrace his weight-loss philosophy. In fact, support for Atkins's approach has only come in recent years.

The details of the program that Dr. Atkins espoused in the 1970s are considerably different from the recommendations found in his most recent book. Early on he advocated eating large amounts of meats and eggs and wasn't fond of any carbohydrates, even vegetables. Dr. Atkins's program evolved over the past 30 years as new research revealed the problems with eating saturated fats, the health benefits of eating 5 to 10 servings daily of vegetables, and the creation of the glycemic index. In fact, in his most recent books, Dr. Atkins included a glycemic index list and advised his readers to eat low glycemic.

We're giving you some information on the Atkins approach so that you can understand the differences between his program and your glycemic index weight-loss program. We don't recommend the Atkins approach. Eating based on the glycemic index gives you excellent results without an induction phase or eating unbalanced meals.

Today's Atkins program includes the following features:

- Begins with a two-week induction phase limiting carbs to two cups of free vegetables and one serving of other low-glycemic vegetables per day.

- Puts a person into ketosis during the induction phase.

- Adds back only five grams of carbs per day per week during the ongoing weight-loss program.

- Recommends eating low-glycemic carbs over high-glycemic carbs in the maintenance phase.

- Strongly urges the dieter to avoid caffeine and the artificial sweetener aspartame.

You don't need a three-phase program to lose weight. In fact, you don't need to go into ketosis to lose weight. And we know that your body needs more vegetables than allowed on this program.

What the Program Misses. Dr. Atkins's program gives comprehensive advice about which kinds of carbohydrates to eat and how to eat them, but it falls short in the following areas:

◆ It ignores the fact that high stress levels can cause weight gain and prevent weight loss.

◆ It is too strict with free foods. These have virtually no glycemic load and they don't need to be restricted. A person isn't permitted to eat 5 to 10 servings of vegetables and fruits during the induction phase, and perhaps not even during the ongoing phase.

The Atkins program missing the mark in these areas probably explains why some dieters fail to lose weight on the program or fail to keep it off. The glycemic index weight-loss program takes all these factors into account so that you get the results you want.

The South Beach Diet

The South Beach Diet Supercharged: Faster Weight Loss and Better Health for Life

The original South Beach Diet was a stunning success and this follow-up book offers an updated version of the original three-phase program along with an all new three-phase exercise program.

The South Beach Diet Supercharged by Arthur Agatston M.D., and Joseph Signorile offers a weight-loss program that incorporates the latest research on the wisdom of eating certain foods, such as good fats, low-glycemic carbohydrates, and lean meats. Next, the maintenance phase is totally flexible, allowing you to eat high-glycemic carbs and even junk foods, provided that you don't start gaining weight.

The three-phase eating plan in phases one and two is problematic. You may not eat enough total calories to keep your metabolism stoked and you aren't eating enough bulk or fiber at each meal. The maintenance plan seems to get confused and doesn't continue advocating eating mostly low-glycemic carbohydrates. The well-intended premise is that by the time you reach phase three, your eating preferences are reformed, and you'll only want to eat the healthiest foods, including low-glycemic carbs. This is wishful thinking, because many dieters are longing to return to their old eating habits.

We applaud the new focus on exercise because it helps with weight loss and is a necessary part of being a vibrant and healthy person.

D

Glycemic Index Resources and Support

Look here for resources that support your glycemic index weight-loss program. We've included information for exercising and supplements, as well as books and websites that will further your knowledge about the glycemic index.

Exercise

Back Roller. Use for relaxation, back alignment, detoxification, and stress reduction. Purchase at www.amazon.com.

Body Rolling (www.yamunabodyrolling.com). Purchase the book *The Ultimate Body Rolling Workout* and the balls. Use to flatten your tummy, reduce cellulite, and ease stress.

Collage Video (www.collagevideo.com). From yoga to Pilates to kickboxing, you can find DVDs and videos on just about any exercise method. At the site, you'll find short video clips of every video, so you can check them out before you purchase. You can build a comprehensive home library from which to select the type of workout that suits your mood or energy level each day.

Fitballs (www.balldynamics.com). Improve your core strength, balance, flexibility, and posture by using resistant exercise balls. This site offers video exercise programs and books that show you how.

Gaiam.com. Use this catalog and Internet-based shopping site for Pilates, yoga, and natural health solutions.

Pilates exercise (www.Stottpilates.com). On this site you'll find information about Pilates exercise as well as videos, equipment, and a listing of Stott-certified instructors in the United States and Canada. You can find many other websites with Pilates information. To find a studio near you, use the Yellow Pages. Another excellent website is http://pilates.about.com/.

Stretching, **by Bob Anderson and Jean Anderson**. Shelter Publications, 2004. This book shows you the correct postures to improve flexibility and reduce stress while increasing energy through stretching.

Your local fitness center may offer exercise classes, aerobic-training equipment, and strength-training machines. Some have lap-swimming pools, racquetball courts, basketball, and tennis courts. Some fitness centers that are funded by local cities and counties are low in price and offer excellent classes and instruction.

Glycemic Index Lists

www.glycemicindex.com. This website is sponsored by the University of Sydney in Australia and contains valuable information on the glycemic index. You can find the glycemic index of individual carbohydrates. The website is based on the research and books of Jennie Brand-Miller, one of the originators of the glycemic index.

www.mendosa.com. The author of this site, David Mendosa, has done a terrific job of building an informative and interesting website that features information on the glycemic index. He includes a complete glycemic index listing of every food tested and includes the glycemic load as well.

Glycemic Index and Glycemic Load Computer Software

GlycoLoad (www.phelpsteam.com/glycoload). This downloadable software costs about $16. You'll find listings for all tested carbohydrates. An added benefit is that the software program automatically computes the glycemic load of each food based on your serving size.

www.mendosa.com. Print or download a comprehensive glycemic index list with glycemic load for standard-size servings from this site. Free.

Supplements

Electrolyte-balancing supplements—Emergen-C electrolyte-balance packets come in many flavors and are widely available at grocery and health-food stores. They contain 32 mineral complexes plus plenty of magnesium, potassium, and B vitamins. Mix in hot or cold water and enjoy. They fizz and can be added to sparkling mineral water or diluted fruit juice. Emergen-C offers a powerful energy boost for the late-afternoon blahs or after strenuous exercise. Use Emergen-C in place of sports electrolyte drinks that contain sugar and high-fructose corn syrup.

Greens Plus—Mix a tablespoon of this green powder in a glass of water. Contains a plethora of antioxidants that help alkalize your body's acid/alkaline balance. Helpful for yeast infections and to decrease sugar cravings. Available online at www.greensplus. com, www.vitaminshoppe.com, or your local health-food store.

Fish oil—Take 1-2 tablespoons per day. Carlson's Fish Oil is lemon-flavored and tastes great. Find at www.vitaminshoppe.com or at your local health-food store. You can also take about 5 capsules of fish oil a day, either regular or enteric coated.

Psyllium—A fiber supplement that aids in regular elimination and also helps you consume an adequate amount of dietary fiber daily. Contains no calories or sweeteners. Take as directed, then follow with one more glass of water. Widely available in bulk at health-food stores.

Fennel-seed tea—Lower anxiety levels and use as a digestive aid. Especially great for bloated or gassy stomachs. Steep 1 teaspoon of fennel seed in a mug of hot water. You'll find the best price by purchasing in bulk at a health-food store rather than by shopping the spice aisle of the grocery store.

Cortisol-lowering supplements—The following supplements can help you lower your levels of cortisol. We don't advise taking all of them at once—you probably don't need all of them. Start with B vitamins. Then add the others if you need more support from time to time.

- ◆ **B vitamins**—Aid in reducing stress levels. When your body is stressed, it uses them up quickly and needs more. Purchase a high-stress B vitamin complex from your health-food store.

- **Liquid B₁₂**—Put a dropper-full under your tongue and you'll find that your stress levels decrease. Widely available at health-food stores.

- **L-Theanine**—This is the soothing component in black or green tea and is widely available in capsules at health-food stores.

Websites

Check out these websites: www.iVillage.com and body.aol.com/diet-fitness. They offer up-to-the-minute weight-loss information on everything you can think of: exercise, fat tummies, glycemic index, scientific research, foods, vitamins, recipes. What makes these sites so valuable is that they're updated frequently and are easily accessible.

When you're browsing these sites, you'll find something more than just information. They have a way of subtly encouraging you to be successful. The underlying message is bright, cheerful, and energetic. The web designers have done a masterful job of inviting you to return over and over again for fun, support, and a daily dose of *joie de vive*.

When you're tempted to toss in the towel or to binge on white, fluffy, or sticky carbs, visit one of these sites. You could empower yourself to turn around your mental attitude.

Glycemic Index Weight-Loss Menus

We've included menu suggestions for you as you embark on your glycemic index weight loss program. Menu items with asterisk (*) have accompanying recipes in Appendix F.

If you are eating on the Keep It Simple Program, you can modify the menus by omitting the wheat products and instead adding more vegetables—but not white potatoes, which are high glycemic.

You need to eat more than 1,400–1,500 calories a day if you are very physically active. If so, you can add a low-glycemic snack or two from the list here:

- 1 piece of fresh fruit and 12 nuts

- 2 cups vegetables with 1 oz. hard cheese

- 1 cup raw vegetables with ¼ cup hummus

- 1–2 cups vegetable soup

- 1 cup winter squash with cinnamon, sprinkled with stevia with FOS

- 1 cup celery sticks with ½ TB. peanut butter

- 2 cups cucumber and onion slices with ½ TB. sour cream or ¼ cup avocado dip

♦ 1 large green pepper and 1 large red pepper, sliced, with 1 oz. cheddar cheese

♦ 2 TB. cashews and vinegar over 2 cups raw tomato and zucchini slices

Keep It Simple—Day 1

Breakfast

Eggplant Chicken*; 1 cup

Fresh peach slices; ½ cup

Fresh blueberries; ½ cup

Lunch

Turkey Quesadilla Plate* with ½ cup sliced vegetables

Fresh pear or apple; 1 large

Snack

Dark chocolate bar; 1.5 oz

Herbal tea

Dinner

Grilled salmon; 3 oz

Fresh vegetable salad; 2 cups (spinach, tomatoes, cucumbers, onions, carrots, broccoli)

Vinaigrette salad dressing; 2 TB

Corn on cob; 1 small ear

Olive oil, or butter; 1 tsp

Keep It Simple—Day 2

Breakfast

Quick Denver Omelet with Salsa*; one-half recipe with 2 eggs

Fresh pineapple; 1 cup, cubed

Lunch

Grape, Garbanzo Bean, and Nut Salad; ⅓ cup grapes, ⅓ cup garbanzo beans, and ~10 nuts

Grilled chicken; 3 oz

Salad dressing; 2 TB

Snack

Ginger Avocado Dip*; ½ cup

Jicama and raw carrots; 2 cups

Dinner

Grilled halibut; 4 oz

Butter or olive oil; 2 tsp.

Steamed broccoli; 1 cup

Roasted beets with herbs; 1 cup

Baked Apple with Almonds*; 1 apple

Comprehensive–Day 1

Breakfast

Whole-wheat breakfast burrito; 1 high-fiber whole-wheat tortilla

Grilled chicken; 3 oz

Southwestern Gazpacho*; ½ cup

Cheddar cheese; ½ oz

Fresh mango slices; 1 cup

Lunch

Green Apple, Spinach, and Walnut Tuna Salad; 1 apple, 2 cups spinach, 4 walnut halves, 1 can tuna with 2 tsp. salad dressing

Stone-ground whole-wheat bread; 1 slice

Cream cheese; 1 TB

Snack

Raw veggies; 1 cup

Hummus*; ½ cup

Dinner

Pork Chops with Oranges*; 1 chop

Sweet potatoes with Parmesan cheese; ½ cup potato and 1 TB cheese

Fresh green beans; 2 cups

Comprehensive—Day 2

Breakfast

Almond Cinnamon Oatmeal with Berries*; 1 cup oatmeal and 1 cup berries

Low-fat cottage cheese; ¾ cup

Whole raw almonds; ~6

Lunch

Crab Soup with Red Bell Pepper*; 2 cups

Whole-grain Wasa crackers with mozzarella cheese; 2 crackers and 1 oz. cheese

Kiwi slices on lettuce leaf; ½ cup kiwi

Snack

Fresh apple; 1 large

Salted cashews; ~12

Herbal tea

Dinner

Beef Stir-Fry with Vegetables*; 2 cups

Whole-grain basmati rice; ½ cup

Dark chocolate; 1 oz

Low-Glycemic Recipes

We've created these recipes to give you a starting place for cooking delicious low-glycemic foods. The cooking methods are the same used in most cookbooks. But you'll be using different ingredients—less white flour and sugar, more farm-sourced foods, and perhaps many more vegetables and fruit.

The recipes are nutritionally designed to give you balanced meals of proteins, carbohydrates, and fat. You'll find more low-glycemic recipes in our cookbook, *The Complete Idiot's Guide Glycemic Index Cookbook*.

Bon appétit.

Breafast

Saturday Eggs

Eggs poached in heavy cream and topped with nutmeg and cheddar cheese.

Yields 4 eggs in cream
Prep time: 5 minutes
Cook time: 10 minutes
Serving size: 1 egg in cream
Each serving:
glycemic index: 0 very low
glycemic load: 0
calories: 148
protein: 8 g
animal protein: 8 g
vegetable protein: 0 g
carbohydrates: 0 g
fiber: 0 g
fat: 12g
saturated fat: 7 g

2 tsp. butter

¼ cup heavy cream

4 eggs

1 TB. shredded cheddar cheese

⅛ tsp. nutmeg

1. Heat butter in a small skillet over medium-low heat. Gently pour in cream. Break eggs into the pan on top of cream.

2. Gently baste eggs with cream until eggs are cooked through. Sprinkle with cheese and let melt slightly. Sprinkle with nutmeg.

Body of Knowledge

These eggs are very low glycemic and rich in fat. Dietary fat increases appetite satisfaction and extends the flavor of food. You may find that a one-egg serving of Saturday Eggs is plenty and all you need. Add fruit such as berries or melon to complete this meal.

Monterey Jack Frittata

An easy top-of-the-stove egg pie with tomatoes and spinach.

4 eggs

½ cup cooked lean meat or chicken

4 TB. shredded Parmesan cheese

1 TB. butter

½ cup chopped fresh tomatoes

½ cup chopped fresh spinach

¼ cup shredded Monterey Jack cheese

Yields one frittata
Prep time: 10 minutes
Cook time: 10 minutes
Serving size: ⅙ frittata
Each serving:
glycemic index: 19 low
glycemic load: <1
calories: 136
protein: 11 g
animal protein: 10 g
vegetable protein: 1 g
carbohydrates: 2 g
fiber: <1 g
fat: 10g
saturated fat: 5 g

1. Whisk eggs in a bowl. Stir in meat or chicken and Parmesan cheese.

2. Melt butter in a skillet over medium heat. Add vegetables and cook until slightly tender, about 5 minutes. Reduce heat and add egg mixture.

3. Cover and cook without stirring for 3 to 5 minutes or until egg is set. Sprinkle shredded Monterey Jack cheese over egg mixture and cover for 1 minute to let cheese melt. Remove from heat and serve.

THIN -couragement

This recipe encourages substitutions. You can use ham, zucchini, cheddar cheese, and vegetables you have on hand.

Quick Denver Omelet with Salsa

Salsa is a garnish to this classic "Denver" omelet with ham, tomatoes, onions, and green peppers.

Yields 4 egg omelet
Prep time: 10 minutes
Cook time: 5 minutes
Serving size: 1 egg plus ¼ filling
Each serving:
glycemic index: 12 very low
glycemic load: <1
calories: 115
protein: 9 g
animal protein: 8 g
vegetable protein: 1 g
carbohydrates: 2 g
fiber: <1 g
fat: 8 g
saturated fat: 3 g

4 eggs

2 tsp. butter

2 TB. diced ham

2 TB. diced green pepper

2 TB. diced tomatoes

2 TB. diced onion

¼ cup salsa

1. Whisk eggs in mixing bowl. Heat butter in a skillet over low-medium heat. Pour in eggs and cook until barely set.

2. Sprinkle ham, green pepper, tomatoes, and onion over eggs and cook about 30 seconds. Fold omelet in half and continue to cook until browned on top and creamy inside.

3. Serve with salsa for topping.

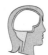 **Body of Knowledge**

Omelets are quicker than you think. Dice the ingredients the night before, and your preparation time in the morning takes as long as brewing a pot of coffee.

Appetizers

Ginger Avocado Dip

A different flavor for the avocado—this time with an Asian influence.

2 fresh avocados

1 TB. lemon juice

¼ cup fruit preserves (or orange marmalade)

1 tsp. minced fresh ginger

Sliced fruit and vegetables

1. Mash avocado gently. Stir in lemon juice, preserves, and ginger.

2. Serve with fresh fruit slices and raw cut-up vegetables.

THIN -couragement

Low-glycemic eating is anything but boring with this unusual dip for vegetables and fruit. Serve it as a topping for eggs and fish, too.

Yields 2 cups dip
Prep time: 10 minutes
Cook time: none
Serving size: ¼ cup dip
Each serving:
glycemic index: 44 low
glycemic load: 5
calories: 52
protein: 1 g
animal protein: 0 g
vegetable protein: 1 g
carbohydrates: 10 g
fiber: 2 g
fat: 5 g
saturated fat: 1 g

Hummus

A favorite garbanzo bean and garlic dip.

Yields 4 ramekins dip
Prep time: 5 minutes
Cook time: About 15 minutes
Serving size: ½ cup dip
Each serving:
glycemic index: 33 low
glycemic load: 6
calories: 260
protein: 10 g
animal protein: 0 g
vegetable protein: 10 g
carbohydrates: 20 g
fiber: 6 g
fat: 12 g
saturated fat: 2 g

1 (14-oz.) can garbanzo beans, drained

4 TB. sesame seed paste

2 tsp. minced garlic

3 TB. lemon juice

2 TB. pine nuts

Dash paprika

Sliced vegetable: red bell peppers.

1. Process beans in a food processor until puréed. Remove to a mixing bowl.

2. Stir in sesame seed paste, garlic, and lemon juice. If needed, add a small amount of water to aid in mixing.

3. To serve, sprinkle with pine nuts and a dash of paprika. Serve with raw vegetables such as sliced red bell peppers for dipping.

 -couragement

Hummus is easy to pack along for snacks. Eat with a spoon, or with rye crackers, fruit, or vegetables. It's high in protein and fiber.

Turkey Quesadilla Plate

Enjoy the taste of a Southwestern quesadilla with refried beans and raw vegetables.

1 (16-oz.) can refried beans

1 cup chopped cooked turkey

2 green onions, sliced

½ cup finely chopped fresh cilantro

1 tomato, finely chopped, and drained

2 tsp. finely chopped, pickled jalapeño peppers

½ cup shredded mozzarella cheese

¼ cup shredded cheddar cheese

Sliced vegetables: jicama, red and green bell pepper, celery sticks.

Yields 3 cups quesadilla mix
Prep time: 15 minutes
Cook time: 15–20 minutes
Serving size: ½ cup quesadilla mix
Each serving:
glycemic index: 46 low
glycemic load: 7
calories: 183
protein: 19 g
animal protein: 14 g
vegetable protein: 5 g
carbohydrates: 17 g
fiber: 7 g
fat: 7g
saturated fat: 3 g

1. Preheat oven to 350°F.

2. Spread refried beans on a 9- or 10-inch pie pan.

3. Evenly distribute turkey, onions, cilantro, tomato, and peppers on beans. Top with cheese.

4. Bake for 15–20 minutes until cheese is melted. Serve with sliced jicama, sliced red and green bell pepper, and celery sticks.

Smoked Salmon Dip with Capers

Smoked salmon with sour cream and capers is the perfect appetizer before a special dinner.

Yields 1½ cup dip
Prep time: 10 minutes
Cook time: none
Serving size: ¼ cup dip
Each serving:
glycemic index: 0 very low
glycemic load: 0
calories: 100
protein: 12 g
animal protein: 12 g
vegetable protein: 0 g
carbohydrates: <1 g
fiber: 0 g
fat: 5.5 g
saturated fat: 2.5 g

4 oz. smoked salmon

½ cup sour cream

½ tsp. minced onion

⅛ tsp. paprika

2 TB. capers

⅛ tsp. freshly ground black pepper

Rye crackers

1. Cut salmon into small pieces in a mixing bowl. Stir in sour cream. Add onion, paprika, capers, and ground black pepper. Blend well.

2. Serve with rye crackers.

-couragement

> This dip is excellent as a side serving for grilled meats and fish. Or serve over greens and vegetables as a main-course salad.

Soups

Southwestern Gazpacho

Fresh and crunchy vegetables blended with spices for a savory starter at a summer lunch or dinner.

1 small jalapeño pepper, stemmed and seeded

1 tsp. minced garlic, cut in 2-inch pieces

2 green onions

1 green pepper, seeded and sliced

1 red bell pepper, seeded and sliced

4 ribs celery, cut in 2-inch pieces

1 cucumber, cut into 2-inch slices

2 ripe tomatoes, cut in half

2 cups tomato juice

3 TB. red wine vinegar

4 shakes Tabasco sauce, or to taste

3 TB. fresh basil, finely chopped

1 tsp. dried oregano

¼ tsp. dried red pepper flakes

1 (4½ oz.) can sliced ripe black olives

1 TB. capers, drained

Yields 4 cups
Prep time: 20 minutes
Cook time: None
Serving size: ¾ cup gazpacho
Each serving:
glycemic index: 38 low
glycemic load: <1
calories: 58
protein: 1 g
animal protein : 0 g
vegetable protein: 1 g
carbohydrates: 5 g
fiber: 1 g
fat: 0 g
saturated fat: 0 g

1. In a food processor, finely chop jalapeño pepper with garlic. Add green onions, green and red peppers, celery, cucumber, and tomatoes and process. Remove mixture from processor and put into a large bowl.

2. Stir in tomato juice, red wine vinegar, Tabasco, basil, oregano, red pepper flakes, black olives, and capers. Chill before serving.

Body of Knowledge

Gazpacho is a cold soup filled with seasonal vegetables, sometimes chopped, and sometimes puréed. You can purée this soup if you prefer and serve with a dollop of sour cream.

Crab Soup with Red Bell Pepper

Mushrooms and tomatoes flavor this hearty main-dish crab soup.

Yields 12 cups soup
Prep time: 15 minutes
Cook time: 45 minutes
Serving size: 2 cups soup
Each serving:
glycemic index: 10 very low
glycemic load: 2
calories: 197
protein: 8 g
animal protein: 7 g
vegetable protein: 1 g
carbohydrates: 14 g
fiber: 5 g
fat: 9 g
saturated fat: 1 g

2 TB. plus 2 TB. olive oil

1 tsp. minced garlic

1 large onion, chopped

3 red bell peppers, cut in 1-inch pieces

2 cups sliced fresh mushrooms

2 quarts water

2 cans crabmeat

2 oz. brandy

2 TB. tomato paste

2 tsp. minced jalapeño peppers

3 TB. chopped parsley

6 Roma tomatoes, cut in quarters

1. Heat 2 tablespoons olive oil in a saucepan. Add garlic and onion and sauté until onion is transparent and soft. Remove onions and garlic.

2. In saucepan, heat remaining 2 tablespoons olive oil and sauté red bell peppers and mushrooms until tender.

3. Add onions and garlic. Stir in water, crabmeat, brandy, tomato paste, jalapeño peppers, parsley, and tomatoes. Bring to a boil and simmer for 15 minutes.

THIN-couragement

If you love mushrooms and crab, you'll enjoy every bite of this low-glycemic soup. Serve with a fresh green salad or vegetable.

Main Dishes

Eggplant Chicken

Garlic and feta cheese lend a Greek flavor to eggplant and shredded chicken breast.

3 TB. olive oil

2 tsp. minced garlic

2 cups fresh sliced eggplant

2 cups cooked shredded chicken breast

2 TB. parsley

½ cup crumbled feta cheese

4 fresh tomatoes, quartered

1. Heat olive oil in skillet. Sauté garlic and eggplant. Add chicken breast and parsley. Heat until warmed throughout.

2. Sprinkle with feta cheese. Serve with tomato wedges.

Body of Knowledge

Eggplant beautifully picks up the flavor and aroma of the garlic, olive oil, and parsley in this recipe.

Yields 4 cups plus tomato wedges
Prep time: 10 minutes
Cook time: 20 minutes
Serving size: 1 cup plus one tomato
Each serving:
glycemic index: 25 low
glycemic load: 7
calories: 220
protein: 28 g
animal protein: 25 g
vegetable protein: 3 g
carbohydrates: 8 g
fiber: 2 g
fat: 13 g
saturated fat: 3.6 g

Beef Stir-Fry with Vegetables

Colorful steamed vegetables brighten this beef stir-fry.

Yields 16 cups
Prep time: 20 minutes
Cook time: 20 minutes
Serving size: 2 cups plus ½ cup rice
Each serving:
glycemic index: 38 low
glycemic load: 8
calories: 302
protein: 22 g
animal protein: 14 g
vegetable protein: 8 g
carbohydrates: 22 g
fiber: 5 g
fat: 9 g
saturated fat: 1.5 g

4 TB. soy sauce

1 TB. cornstarch

1 TB. honey

1 tsp. salt

½ tsp. ground black pepper

2 TB. plus 2 TB. canola oil

1 lb. boneless round steak, cut into strips

1 onions, chopped

3 ribs celery, sliced

2 small zucchini, sliced

2 yellow crookneck squash, sliced

2 green bell peppers, cut in strips

3 carrots, sliced diagonally

1 cup sliced fresh mushrooms

1 cup broccoli florets

4 cups cooked basmati rice

1. Make sauce by combining soy sauce, cornstarch, honey, salt, and pepper in a small bowl.

2. Preheat 2 tablespoons oil in a wok or heavy skillet to medium-high. Add steak strips and onions. Stir-fry until meat is browned, cover and simmer 10 minutes. Remove from pan.

3. Add remaining 2 tablespoons oil to wok or skillet and heat. Add celery, zucchini, squash, green bell peppers, carrots, mushrooms, and broccoli. Stir-fry for 5 minutes, then cover and steam 5 minutes.

4. Return meat and onion to pan. Pour sauce over mixture, stir. Steam about 3 minutes. Should be thickened. Serve over basmati rice.

THIN -couragement

You can't go wrong eating lean meats and nonstarchy vegetables. They taste great with many different sauces and condiments.

Pork Chops with Oranges

Pork chops are flavored with ginger, garlic, and oranges.

6 (4 oz.) lean pork chops, with visible fat removed

2 TB. butter

1 tsp. minced garlic

1 1-inch piece ginger root, diced

2 TB. soy sauce

2 tsp. white wine vinegar

6 orange slices with peel, ⅜ thick

¼ cup chopped peanuts

¼ tsp. ground fresh pepper

Yields 6 pork chops
Prep time: 20 minutes
Cook time: 40 minutes
Serving size: 1 (4-oz.) pork chop
Each serving:
glycemic index: 19 low
glycemic load: <1
calories: 298
protein: 23 g
animal protein: 21 g
vegetable protein: 2 g
carbohydrates: 4 g
fiber: 4 g
fat: 14 g
saturated fat: 5g

1. In a medium-size skillet with tight-fitting lid, brown pork chops in butter. Cover and cook 20 minutes over medium-high heat.

2. Remove cover and chops. Add garlic, ginger root, soy sauce, and vinegar to skillet. Stir. Top with pork chops. Place one orange slice on each chop. Cover and cook 20 minutes until pork is cooked thoroughly.

3. Serve topped with chopped peanuts and pepper.

Wrong Weigh

Don't be afraid of pork being fattening. Remove all visible fat before cooking and then enjoy the succulent orange and ginger-flavored meat.

Cod Fillets in a Spicy Tomato Sauce

The unusual sauce is flavored with fennel, dry mustard, cumin, and turmeric to give the cod a distinctive and exotic taste.

Yields 2 pounds cod plus 1 cup vegetables and sauce
Prep time: 10 minutes
Cook time: 30 minutes
Serving size: 4 ounces cod plus ⅛ vegetables and sauce
Each serving:
glycemic index: 34 low
glycemic load: <1
calories: 140
protein: 29 g
animal protein: 28 g
vegetable protein: 1 g
carbohydrates: 4 g
fiber: <1 g
fat: 4 g
saturated fat: <1 g

2 TB. olive oil

1 small onion, finely chopped

2 cloves garlic, peeled, finely chopped

1 (14-oz.) can chopped tomatoes

¼ tsp. ground turmeric

1 tsp. fennel seeds

1 tsp. dry mustard

½ tsp. ground cumin

¾ tsp. salt

½ tsp. cayenne

2 lbs. cod, cut into fillets

1. In a large skillet, heat olive oil and sauté onion and garlic until translucent.

2. Add tomatoes, turmeric, fennel seeds, dry mustard, cumin, salt, and cayenne. Bring to a boil and simmer gently for 15 minutes.

3. Add fish and simmer for 10 minutes or until it flakes.

Body of Knowledge

Keep these less popular spices and herbs in your spice cabinet. They add color and interesting flavor to vegetables, seafood, and meat. Fennel seeds make a soothing tea—add 1 teaspoon to a mug of boiling water.

Edamame and Wild Rice Salad

Freshly picked and frozen soybeans are dressed with tomatoes, celery, and dressing, and paired with wild rice.

1 (16-oz.) bag frozen, shelled edamame	**1 TB. olive oil**
1 cup cooked wild rice	**1 TB. balsamic vinegar**
1 (15-oz.) can diced tomatoes	**½ tsp. salt**
2 cups chopped celery	**¼ tsp. ground black pepper**
2 TB. chopped green onions	**8 lettuce leaves**

1. Cook edamame according to package directions. Drain and cool.

2. In a large bowl, mix together wild rice, tomatoes, celery, green onions, olive oil, vinegar, salt, and pepper.

3. Add edamame to wild-rice mixture and serve on lettuce leaves.

Body of Knowledge

Edamame are natural unprocessed green, picked fresh soybeans. They're a legume, but served as a vegetable in this recipe.

Yields 8 cups salad

Prep time: 10 minutes

Cook time: 10 minutes

Serving size: 1 cup salad

Each serving:

glycemic index: 33 low

glycemic load: 3

calories: 93

protein: 6 g

animal protein: 0 g

vegetable protein: 6 g

carbohydrates: 9 g

fiber: 3 g

fat: 3 g

saturated fat: <1 g

Desserts

Baked Apples with Almonds

These baked apples fill your home with the fragrant aroma of cinnamon, nutmeg, and cloves.

Yields 4 apples
Prep time: 10 minutes
Cook time: 45 minutes
Serving size: 1 apple
Each serving:
glycemic index: 43 low
glycemic load: 14
calories: 139
protein: 2 g
animal protein: 0 g
vegetable protein: 2 g
carbohydrates: 32 g
fiber: 3 g
fat: 2 g
saturated fat: <1 g

4 tsp. raisins

4 tsp. sliced almonds

1 tsp. cinnamon

Dash nutmeg

Dash ground cloves

4 cooking apples, such as Fuji, McIntosh, Granny Smith, or Jonathan, cored

4 tsp. honey

1. Preheat oven to 375°F.

2. Mix together raisins, almonds, cinnamon, nutmeg, and cloves in a small bowl.

3. Place apples in a baking dish. Fill hollow of each with ¼ raisin mixture. Top each with 1 teaspoon with honey.

4. Bake for 45 minutes. Serve hot or cold.

 -couragement

> Apples satisfy your appetite and provide important nutrients and fiber. "An apple a day …" may not be technically true, but they make for great eating.

Cocoa Granola Bars

The rich taste of chocolate, walnuts, and raisins flavors these granola bars.

2 eggs

2 TB. honey

2 TB. canola oil

1 tsp. vanilla extract

1 cup unprocessed wheat bran

1 cup long-cooking oats

¼ cup coarsely chopped walnuts

¼ cup raisins

¼ cup unsweetened cocoa powder

½ cup chocolate morsels

Yields 3 cups bars
Prep time: 15 minutes
Cook time: 20 minutes plus 30–40 minutes stand time.
Serving size: ½ cup bar
Each serving:
glycemic index: 42 low
glycemic load: 14
calories: 280
protein: 8 g
animal protein: 0 g
vegetable protein: 8 g
carbohydrates: 25 g
fiber: 7 g
fat: 11 g
saturated fat: 3 g

1. Preheat oven to 325°F.

2. Whisk eggs with honey, canola oil, and vanilla extract in small bowl.

3. Combine wheat bran, oats, walnuts, raisins, cocoa powder, and chocolate morsels. Stir egg mixture into dry ingredients.

4. Flatten mixture on a cookie sheet. For a crisper granola, spread mixture thinly.

5. Bake for 20 minutes. Turn oven off and keep crackers in the oven for an additional 30 to 40 minutes.

-couragement

You don't need to give up chocolate or even your love for chocolate to be at your ideal size. Eat it in low-medium-glycemic recipes and you'll have your chocolate make you thin.

Chocolate Cookies

The pecan flour gives these cookies a rich chocolaty flavor.

Yields 2 dozen cookies
Prep time: 15 minutes
Cook time: 10–15 minute
Serving size: 1 cookies
Each serving:
glycemic index: 17 low
glycemic load: 1.5
calories: 87
protein: 2g
animal protein: 0 g
vegetable protein: 2 g
carbohydrates: 5 g
fiber: 1 g
fat: 8 g
saturated fat: 3 g

1¼ cups pecans, coarsely chopped

½ cup butter

⅓ cup fructose

1 tsp. molasses

1 egg

¼ cup unsweetened cocoa powder

½ tsp. vanilla extract

¼ tsp. salt

1. Preheat oven to 350°F.

2. Process pecans in food processor until they become ground as a flour.

3. In mixer, cream butter with fructose and molasses. Beat in egg. Add cocoa powder, vanilla extract, and salt. Slowly fold in pecan flour and mix to a stiff dough.

4. Form dough into 24 balls and place balls on an ungreased cookie sheet about 1 inch apart. Flatten slightly. Bake for 10–15 minutes.

Body of Knowledge

Eat medium- or high-glycemic foods with a meal, not apart from a meal, and you'll effectively lower the glycemic impact of the food. This works for small amounts of medium- or high-glycemic foods. Too much food is always too much food, no matter what the glycemic index.

Index

C

G

T

NEW from Lucy Beale and
Joan Clark-Warner, M.S., R.D., C.D.E.

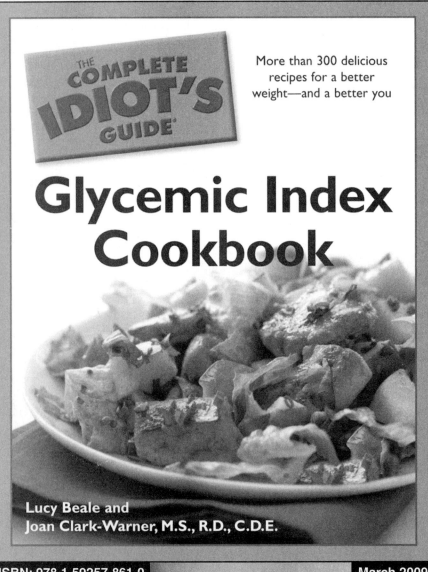

THE COMPLETE IDIOT'S GUIDE

More than 300 delicious
recipes for a better
weight—and a better you

Glycemic Index Cookbook

Lucy Beale and
Joan Clark-Warner, M.S., R.D., C.D.E.

ISBN: 978-1-59257-861-0

March 2009